Bile Salts in Health and Disease

TO SUNE BERGSTRÖM
who more than anyone got
bile salts moving

BILE SALTS
IN HEALTH AND DISEASE

K. W. HEATON
M.D., M.R.C.P.

Senior Lecturer in Medicine, University of Bristol
Department of Medicine, Bristol Royal Infirmary

CHURCHILL LIVINGSTONE
EDINBURGH AND LONDON
1972

First published 1972

International Standard Book Number
0 443 00917 1

Printed in Great Britain by
The Whitefriars Press Ltd., London and Tonbridge

Contents

Acknowledgements

I am indebted to many people who have made this book possible: firstly colleagues with whom I have been privileged to work, Drs. Warren Austad, Leon Lack, Mal Tyor, John Morris, Tom Low-Beer, Ru Pomare and most importantly my wife Susan; secondly, a superb typist Linda Savage; thirdly, an ever helpful department of medical illustration, headed by Mr. John Eatough.

I am grateful for permission to reproduce figures to Dr. Alan Hofmann, Dr. Donald Small, Dr. Ian Bouchier and Dr. James Gregg.

Foreword

Professor ALAN E. READ, M.D., F.R.C.P.
Professor of Medicine in the University of Bristol

Though it is often said that the major advances in medical science will in the future stem from the scientist rather than the clinician, it is still true, however, that it is the clinician who must sift and apply such new discoveries for the welfare of his patients. One field of interest which closely involves both scientist and clinician is that of bile salt metabolism. It is perhaps rather surprising that knowledge about these compounds has been so long in reaching any fruition, but one must blame various things, including difficulty in obtaining samples of bile under physiological conditions, the availability of suitable labelled compounds, the difficulty associated with biochemical techniques, etc.

We, the clinicians, have thus been presented over the past 10 to 15 years with a wealth of scientific information concerning biliary physiology and bile salt metabolism and the problem now seems to be to determine where this information fits into the complex and sometimes seemingly unscientific network of clinical medicine. The task might at first seem overwhelming, the biochemistry is perhaps difficult to understand, the methodology which has been used lies outside that normally part of the clinical approach, and the description of yet another entero-hepatic circulation is enough to chill the staunchest clinical heart!

Dr. K. W. Heaton's monograph is therefore doubly welcome because in a comparatively small space it presents the background to the scientific aspects of bile salt metabolism and draws the attention of the reader to those parts of clinical practice where disordered organ structure and function may be the result of abnormal bile salt metabolism. Some of these aspects, particularly the gastro-intestinal ones, are clear cut and already proven—others set intriguing problems for research in the future, as they involve such important problems as the aetiology of some varieties of cancer and the problems of arterial degenerative disease.

This monograph sets a pattern which others might do well to copy. Its aim is a thoroughly proper one, namely the application of science to the welfare of the sick patient. Perhaps it will be a pattern for the future when, as happens on occasions, the profusion of scientific fact in any one field seems to overwhelm the apparent paucity of clinical application. Dr. Heaton is to be congratulated on his efforts to direct the flow of information between the interested parties in this important field of research. In so doing he has provided a considerable service for clinicians of many disciplines, including specialists in gastroenterology, arterial disease, and lipid metabolism. In return it would be worthwhile inviting the scientists concerned to come out of their narrow specialties and see what has happened and what can possibly be predicted because of new knowledge in a variety of clinical situations.

Both scientists and clinicians have contributed to the substance of this book—both groups should be encouraged to read it. It deserves success.

1   Historical Perspective

This chapter originally appeared in *Journal of the Royal College of Physicians of London,* **6**(1), 83-97, and is reproduced here by kind permission of the Editor.

Since antiquity, bile has been regarded as both important and potentially dangerous. For the greater part of recorded history it has in fact dominated man's concepts of health and disease. The ancient Greeks, probably at the time of Pythagoras in the sixth century BC [586], evolved the doctrine of the four humours or body fluids, and this theory governed medical thinking until the rebirth of science in the sixteenth and seventeenth centuries. The four humours were yellow bile, black bile, blood, and mucus or phlegm. A balanced mixture of the humours (*krasis*) was the basis of health, and disease resulted when there was an imbalance (*dyskrasis*) due to excess of one member. Each humour had clearly defined elemental properties and was associated with a specific temperament. Yellow or bitter bile, being the humoral equivalent of the element Fire, was regarded as responsible for the heat of the body and as having potent drying qualities. Its influence accounted for a choleric temperament. Black bile, which was cold and dry like Earth, was the basis of a melancholic spirit (Greek, *melas,* black, *khole,* bile). Thus, to this day our speech bears traces of the humoral doctrine. Yellow bile was what we still call bile, but black bile was at first a philosophical abstraction and later identified with the blood in the splenic vein.

The reason that the ancients considered bile so important was probably its strikingly bitter taste as well as its strong colour. Having only their unaided senses to guide them in their investigations of the body and its diseases they must have been impressed by the fact that bile is the only body fluid that tastes bitter. Many centuries later men still marvelled that 'one Drop of it will make a whole Pint of Water bitter' [11]. Even today, a particularly bitter disappointment is referred to as a galling experience and a popular Christmas Carol includes the

words 'The holly bears a bark as bitter as any gall'. The bitter taste of
bile is due to its content of bile salts, so it can be said that bile salts
greatly influenced men's thinking long before they were 'discovered' in
the early nineteenth century.

EARLY IDEAS ABOUT BILE AS EXCRETORY MATERIAL

Early writers stressed the acrid, irritant nature of bile and it was this,
no doubt, that led Aristotle, in the fourth century BC, to dismiss it,
according to Gibson [220], 'as a mere excrement, and of no other use
than by its acrimony to promote the excretion of the Guts'. This view
of bile as nothing but an excretion product was endorsed by Galen, in
the second century AD. Indeed, Galen's theory that the function of the
liver was to convert absorbed nutrients into blood led inevitably to the
concept that bile was the waste-product of this important process. The
only useful function he allowed to bile was aiding the excretion of the
faeces [142]. Galenical teachings held sway for 1,500 years. Thus, in
the sixteenth century Vesalius wrote of bile as 'the thinner refuse of the
liver', which 'with its biting quality irritates the intestines for propelling
this refuse [of the stomach]' [397]. Similarly, Realdus Colombus
[107], the noted anatomist of Cremona, wrote 'bile is discharged from
the gallbladder and carried into the intestines to excite their activity
and . . . compel them to excrete the faeces'.

THE REALISATION OF THE DIGESTIVE ROLE OF BILE

The explosion of scientific knowledge in the seventeenth century
resulted in a radical rethinking of the nature and functions of bile. Two
discoveries were of particular importance. First, Harvey's discovery of
the circulation of the blood rendered untenable the Galenical belief
that the liver is the organ that makes blood and sends it out through the
veins to all parts of the body. Secondly, the discovery of the lacteal
lymph vessels and their drainage via the thoracic duct into the
subclavian vein showed that absorbed nutrients do not necessarily go
straight into the liver. With the collapse of Galen's theory came the
obvious but exciting implication that bile formation was the major
function of the liver. In the words of the English anatomist Gibson
[220], 'so bulky a Bowel was never made for the separation of a mere
excrement'. Gibson argued that, since liver injuries and diseases have

serious consequences, 'that liquor which it separates must have some noble use, and such as is very necessary unto life'. The Dutch anatomist, Diemerbroek, was the chief protagonist of this revolutionary concept of bile, but so strong was the influence of Galen and Aristotle that his views were by no means universally accepted. Thus, the famous English anatomist Francis Glisson [222] wrote of bile, 'It is also nauseous, corrosive and noxious to all organs, especially by its heat and dryness . . . No advantage at all, but the greatest damage results if it stays for a long time in the body. Thus I conclude that it is by no means a nutritious [= digestive], but solely an excrementitious fluid'.

The new function ascribed to bile was to be a 'ferment for the Chyle'. Diemerbroek recognised that bile mixes 'with the alimentary mass concocted in the stomach, . . . which it causes to ferment'. He went on to suggest that, 'it dissolves and separates the thinner parts of the chyle from the thicker ones, and attenuates them so much that they may easily be taken up by the narrow orifices of the lacteal vessels'. This theory is remarkably near the modern view of the main digestive function of bile being the reduction of particle size.

The idea that the special role of bile is to aid fat digestion was clearly put forward in the 18th century. Physicians like John Arbuthnot [11] and Thomas Coe [104] noticed that ordinary folk were using ox bile as an alternative to soap for washing clothes, and that it was particularly effective for removing grease marks. Furthermore, painters had long used it to help mix their colours. Arbuthnot reasonably concluded that bile is 'a saponaceous substance and . . . mixeth the oily and watery Parts of the Aliment together'. Physicians, with their usual pragmatism, were quick to recognise bile as a 'Natural Digestive' [25], and as 'an animal soap' [77]. They pointed out that bile is stored in the gallbladder for use at meal times, and is discharged high up in the intestine, and, also, that obvious ill-effects accompany its deficiency in the bowel, which 'plainly show it is not an useless fluid, but is designed for very important purposes in the animal oeconomy' [104]. On the other hand, anatomists, physiologists, and chemists remained sceptical, perhaps because they were more indoctrinated with the tenacious remnants of Galenical teaching. As late as 1843, Liebig's famous textbook of biochemistry, *Animal Chemistry,* which incidentally devoted more space to bile than to blood, did not so much as hint that bile had a digestive role. Rather, Liebig held that bile was the means of excretion of carbonaceous tissue breakdown products and stated, 'It is obvious that the elements of bile serve for respiration and for the production of animal heat', an amazingly clear echo of the humoral doctrine. Even more remarkably, scientists continued till the present century to discuss the idea that bile is solely an excretion [444].

Attempts to prove by direct experiment that bile has digestive functions did not begin until the nineteenth century. Some crude but significant observations were made by Beaumont [26] in the course of his experiments on Alexis St Martin, the long-suffering young French-Canadian with a post-traumatic gastric fistula. Beaumont mixed olive oil or cream with gastric juice and noted that more fat was dispersed when the juice was strongly bile-stained than when it was clear. He inferred from this and other experiments that bile 'is not commonly necessary for the digestion of food, but . . . when oily food has been used, bile assists its digestion'. The crucial evidence, however, came from experiments in which bile was prevented from entering the intestine. Possibly the earliest of these studies was that of Brodie who tied the common bile duct of an animal and noted the thoracic duct lymph to be thin and depleted of fat [77], but the really conclusive experiment was the creation of a fistula from the gallbladder or common bile duct to the skin, that allowed the entire biliary output to be diverted. Using this technique Schwann [574], Schellbach [559], and particularly Bidder and Schmidt [45], showed that, deprived of bile, a dog would lose weight in spite of a ravenous appetite, and that its faeces were bulky, pale and malodorous and contained a great excess of fat. These classic demonstrations of steatorrhoea proved so finally that bile is important in fat digestion that it is hard to believe that Claude Bernard [42] held for a time to the contrary view. Probably he was misled by his famous discovery that in the rabbit, whose pancreatic duct enters the intestine below the bile duct, only those mesenteric lymphatics that originate below the pancreatic duct orifice become milky after feeding.

THE DISCOVERY OF BILE SALTS

As the argument about the functions of bile reached its climax, the chemists were busy investigating the nature of this enigmatic fluid. Berzelius [44] was apparently the first to recognise the presence of an acid fraction. Gmelin [223], in a more extensive fractionation of ox bile, identified both sodium cholate and taurine, while Demarcay [138] showed that what he called choleic acid (Choleinsäure) was the major solid component of bile. The term bile acid was coined by Liebig [395]. By 1855 it was recognised that glycocholic and taurocholic acids are separate entities and that bile salts are responsible for keeping cholesterol in solution in bile [385].

THE ENTEROHEPATIC CIRCULATION: ITS DISCOVERY AND CHARACTERISATION

Another major development of the mid-nineteenth century was the proof that bile salts undergo an enterohepatic circulation. It had long been suspected that a major portion of bile is absorbed and re-utilised. As far back as the seventeenth century Joseph Borellus, Professor of Mathematics at Naples, had calculated that the total amount of bile entering the duodenum each day was seventeen times the amount of bile present in the biliary tree at any one time and had inferred that 'there is a particular circulation of the bile through the abdomen, performed by the Venae mesaraicae into the trunk of the Porta, thence to the liver, thence through the bilious vessels into the Duodenum to return again by the Mesaraick Veins' [220]. This novel and controversial idea was developed by Edward Barry, Professor of Physic in Dublin, who realised that such a circulation could effect important economies in what he saw as 'the most concocted Humour [= complicated fluid] in the body'. In 1759 wrote: 'It is likewise more than probable, that the more acrid, and active Parts of the Bile, which remain dissolved in the Intestines, after the Chyle has passed the Lacteals, are likewise received into the Meseraic Veins, which . . . soon return again, by this short Circulation, to the Liver; and by these Means supply it with active, genuine Materials, fit for the more easy Preparation, and Secretion of new Bile' [25]. This intuitive description of the enterohepatic circulation is astonishingly accurate, but it was not fully confirmed for another 180 years.

The first solid evidence that part of the bile is reabsorbed was provided by the analyses of Berzelius, Liebig, Pettenkofer and others who showed that, in the absence of diarrhoea, the stools contain insignificant quantities of bile products [613, 395, 384]. Liebig thought that the reabsorbed bile was metabolised and excreted in the breath, others that it was voided in the urine [559]. Credit must be given to Hoffman [299] for wondering about some kind of circulation but it was Hoppe-Seyler who, in 1863 postulated a continuous recirculation of bile salts. This theory received support from the work of Schiff [563] who placed bile in a dog's stomach and noticed within 15 minutes an increased flow of bile and output of bile salts from a biliary fistula. Schiff rightly argued that the choleresis was due to the secretion of the absorbed bile salts, but his views were strongly opposed. His critics were at last silenced by ingenious experiments in which a 'foreign' bile salt was fed to an animal and subsequently identified in its bile. For example, Weiss [693] fed glycocholic acid to dogs, whose bile salts are normally all taurine-conjugated, and demonstrated that the ensuing bile secretion contained 25 to 30 per cent of glycine conjugates. Similarly, Schiff himself [564] took guinea-pigs, whose bile is normally negative to the Pettenkofer test, and by feeding them ox bile made them secrete its contained Pettenkofer-positive bile salts.

These experiments proved the existence of an enterohepatic circulation, but it was left to twentieth-century investigators to demonstrate its economic importance, frequency and efficiency. Whipple and Smith [697] showed the disparity between what the liver can produce unaided and what it normally secretes with the help of recycled material, when they found that the daily bile salt secretion of a bile-fistula dog was eight times greater if the drained bile was returned to the animal than if it was removed. This figure agrees well with modern estimates based on isotopic labelling [306, 279]. Early attempts to calculate the frequency of recirculation in man gave estimates of three cycles daily [343]. The present estimate of two to three cycles per meal still rests mainly on intestinal intubation studies done in the nineteen-fifties by Borgström et al. [59]. Early endeavours to measure the efficiency of recirculation were made in dogs by Schmidt et al. [565] and in hogs by Irvin et al. [330]. Using the amount of duodenally administered bile salt that could be recovered from a cannula in the common bile duct, both groups estimated that about 10 per cent of the bile salts were lost. More accurate radioactive tracer techniques have subsequently shown average wastage per cycle in man to be nearer 3 per cent [306, 279]. Precise measurement of the size of the circulating bile salt pool also had to await radioactive techniques, as did studies of the factors affecting the pool size. Although the existence of a dynamic equilibrium between synthesis and excretion was realised in 1941 by Berman et al., the nature of the homeostatic mechanism is still under very active investigation.

THE INTESTINAL ABSORPTION OF BILE SALTS

The question of the site and route of intestinal absorption of bile salts excited remarkably little interest until the nineteen-sixties. Up till that time it was generally assumed that bile salts were absorbed together with fat in the upper small intestine, unless one excepts the strangely prescient remark of Barry [25] (see page 5). It is true that in 1878 Tappeiner had injected solutions of taurocholate and glycocholate into tied-off loops of dog intestine and shown that absorption was absent from the duodenum, that only glycocholate disappeared from the jejunum but that both bile salts were absorbed from the ileum. However, he did not understand the significance of his data and they attracted no attention. In 1936, Frölicher repeated Tappeiner's experiments in rats and obtained similar results, but again their importance was not realised. The same investigation was to be done a third time [21] before Lack and Weiner in 1961 at last provided the explanation by demonstrating the presence in the ileum of a specialised active transport system for bile salt absorption. Subsequent work has confirmed that the ileum is the major site of bile salt absorption in man as well as in every species of animal or bird tested [691, 145]. Recent work makes it likely that significant absorption of deconjugated bile acids can occur from the colon [548, 427, 453] and under pathological circumstances from the jejunum [148, 298]. The role of the jejunum in absorption of conjugated bile salts remains controversial [298, 411]. As for the route taken by bile salts from the intestine to the liver, the portal vein always seemed the most likely and this was proved by Josephson and Rydin in 1936.

THE ORIGIN, CHEMICAL NATURE, AND METABOLISM OF BILE SALTS

Modern ideas about the origin, chemical nature and metabolism of bile salts derive almost entirely from work done in the last forty years. It was previously assumed that bile salts were made by the liver, if only because they were virtually impossible to detect in body fluids other than the bile. Direct evidence for this belief was the finding that hepatectomised dogs had no bile acids in their blood [613]. Similarly, Smyth and Whipple [611] found that the bile acid secretion of bile fistula dogs fell when liver poisons such as chloroform and phosphorus were administered. Their chemical origin was thought at first to be tissue metabolites; for example, Smith and Whipple [610] considered bile salts to be derived from body and food protein. Chemical analysis showed a striking similarity between bile salts and cholesterol, and this was confirmed when Rosenheim and King [540] elucidated the ring structure of the steroid nucleus. This obviously suggested a precursor-product relationship but some authorities continued to deny this [711] on the ground that feeding cholesterol to bile fistula dogs did not increase their bile salt output. The issue was not finally resolved until Bloch *et al.* [49] showed that a dog given deuterium-labelled cholesterol produced labelled bile salts. Thanks to much further work with isotopic materials, a great deal is now known about the complicated process whereby cholesterol is converted in the liver to bile acids. Much of this work has been done in Sweden, and has been summarised by Bergström *et al.* [38], by Danielsson [120], and by Danielsson and Tchen [125].

The Swedes were quick to see how radioactive labelling of bile salts makes it possible to study their fate in the body. In 1953, Bergström *et al.* described the synthesis of carboxyl-^{14}C-labelled bile salts. The same group developed new chromatographic methods using, especially, Celite columns and paper [593], and have gone on to make literally hundreds of important contributions to our understanding of bile salt metabolism. Of particular importance was the discovery that in the intestinal lumen bile salts are extensively degraded by bacteria and that some of the altered bile salts, especially deoxycholate, are absorbed and recirculated [251, 39, 400]. Other important pioneer work done in Sweden included the first accurate estimation of the kinetics of the enterohepatic circulation by Lindstedt [399], the discovery of the negative feedback mechanism controlling hepatic bile salt synthesis [178, 36], the formulation of the concept that active transport of bile salts is the main driving force in bile secretion [617] and the characterisation of the chemical pattern of bile-salts in human bile [331, 596].

THE CONCEPT OF BILE SALTS AS DETERGENTS

The mode of action of bile salts in their main function of lipid absorption has also been elucidated, mainly in the last forty years. In the mid-nineteenth century Strecker [630] and Marcet [424] had shown that fatty acids are dissolved by taurocholate and by whole bile respectively, but further developments came slowly. This may be because in the latter part of the century the accepted theory of fat absorption was that fatty acids, released by the action of pancreatic lipase on neutral fat, were at once turned into soluble sodium salts or soaps, and that these soaps, together with bile salt, emulsified the bulk of the dietary triglyceride which was then absorbed as an emulsion. At the turn of the century this theory came under attack. Moore, of University College, London, pointed out that many fatty acid soaps such as sodium stearate are in fact poorly soluble and themselves require a solvent, and showed that these fatty acids are dispersed by bile, in both the test-tube and the dog intestine, to form a water-clear solution [445]. He then went on to describe the great solubility of lecithin in bile salt solutions and the consequently increased ability of bile salts to dissolve fatty acids [444]. These writings contain the essence of present-day views but their relevance could not be appreciated until the quite recent discovery that a major end-product of pancreatic lipolysis is monoglyceride [199]. Another and more influential attack on the old 'particulate theory' of fat absorption came in 1900 from Pflüger [678]. He rightly doubted whether emulsion droplets could enter the mucosal cell and, going to the other extreme, postulated a complete hydrolysis of triglyceride, with absorption of fatty acids as soaps and in combination with bile salts. This 'lipolytic theory' held the field for over forty years. During this time the role of bile salts was variously interpreted. In 1916, Wieland and Sorge enunciated the choleic acid principle, that fatty acids combine chemically with bile acids to form water-soluble complexes. This idea was generally accepted for twenty-five years although it was based on experiments with an unphysiological substance, free deoxycholic acid. Verzár accepted total lipolysis (while admitting it had not been demonstrated) but rightly argued that at the acid pH of the upper small intestine fatty acids would not be present as soaps [678]. He showed that at this pH, solutions of glycocholate and taurocholate dissolve fatty acids and saw this as the main role of bile salts. Also, to explain the marked disparity between the quantity of fat absorbed and the amount of bile salt available to assist this absorption, he accepted an ingenious turnstile model in which bile salt, after adsorption to the mucosa, transported numerous loads of fatty acid into the interior of the cell before being absorbed itself [206]. This model has a modern counterpart in the concept of bile salts as lipid exchangers [160].

An essential part of the lipolytic theory was the total hydrolysis of dietary triglycerides into glycerol and free fatty acids. This point was strongly disputed in the early years of this century [678, 613]. At last, in 1945, Frazer and Sammons showed conclusively that monoglycerides and even diglycerides are important end-products of pancreatic lipolysis, and this work was soon confirmed by studies using labelled glycerides (e.g. Borgström [54]). Frazer and his colleagues [200] also showed that the most effective emulsifying system likely to arise in the intestinal contents was a triple combination of bile salt, fatty acid, and monoglyceride. This and other evidence led Frazer [198] to put forward his 'partition theory', which was a partial reinstatement of the old particulate theory since it involved absorption of some triglyceride as a fine emulsion stabilised by his triple system. Although this theory is now discredited [57], it had two important new features which have been included in present-day views on fat absorption [307], namely a detergent complex which included monoglyceride and the formation of negatively charged particles. Its main shortcoming was that its end product was a fine emulsion.

Our belief in a micellar solution as the end product of fat digestion springs from the demonstration of a lipid-rich yet water-clear phase in centrifuged intestinal aspirate [157, 56], together with a growing understanding of the mode of action of detergents. The idea that soap solutions contain highly charged colloidal particles or 'micelles' was developed in 1913 by McBain. In 1936, this theory was extended by Hartley who coined the term 'amphipathy' to express the character of a micelle-forming substance as 'the simultaneous presence of separately satisfiable *sym*pathy and *anti*pathy for water', in other words, 'the possession of both feelings'. Hartley suggested that bile salts are amphipathic compounds, and within a few years papers appeared confirming that bile salt solutions had physical features indicating micelle formation [535], [415]. The choleic acid principle was now quietly buried. The fact that effective detergent solutions usually contain a third component, a polar lipid, was stressed by Lawrence [379], and in 1963 Hofmann described the extraordinary solubility of one such polar lipid, monoglyceride, in bile salt solutions, and the consequently enhanced solubility of a non-polar solute (cf. Moore and Parker [444]). These phenomena were shown to be of physiological relevance by the finding that fatty acids and monoglycerides are rapidly taken up by intestinal mucosa from an artificial micella solution, both *in* *vitro* [341] and *in vivo* [60]. It has also been demonstrated that such insoluble substances as cholesterol and fat-soluble vitamins are readily dissolved in and absorbed from micellar solutions [588, 555], which no doubt explains the long-appreciated necessity of bile for their absorption [460, 237]. These and other findings have led to many new insights into the clinical problem of steatorrhoea [304, 305].

THE PURGATIVE PROPERTIES OF BILE SALTS

The purgative properties of bile have been known since antiquity and have been exploited therapeutically right up to the present. Enemas of eel bile were recommended by Boerhaave 1668-1732 [509] while dried ox bile was a popular laxative until the present century. After bile salts were discovered and isolated many workers studied their cathartic action [613] and it was soon realised that bile salts act mainly on the large intestine, by stimulating its motor activity [573]. Bile salts placed in the dog's rectum caused immediate defaecation [262]. The laxative properties of bile salts have resulted in their being included in innumerable nostrums, a recent well-known example being Bile Beans. In the last few years another explanation has been found for this purgative action. Forth *et al.* [197] showed, in rats, that bile salts inhibit the transport of water and sodium by colonic mucosa. Similarly, perfusion studies in man have shown interference with colonic water and electrolyte absorption by both free and conjugated bile salts [427, 429]. It is still a moot point whether this effect of bile salts is a factor in promoting normal defaecation.

THE TOXICITY OF BILE SALTS

Other pharmacological and toxic properties have been extensively investigated in the past [613]. These have included anticoagulant, antiseptic, haemolytic, and cardiac depressant effects. For centuries the toxicity of bile was a popular subject for research, and as recently as 1938 a whole book was devoted to reviewing this subject [324]. Most of these so-called toxic properties are undoubtedly artefacts of the laboratory. Current interest is largely in the effects of bile salts on the small intestinal mucosa. Much previous work with conjugated materials was rendered invalid by the demonstration of Pope *et al.* in 1966 that thorough purification of conjugated bile salts removes most of their inhibitory properties. However, it has been repeatedly confirmed that, at least *in vitro,* free bile acids, especially deoxycholate, inhibit the absorptive process, probably through a general depression of cellular metabolism [135, 144, 23]. There is evidence that free bile acids damage the intestinal mucosa [412]. This effect may be abolished by high concentrations of conjugated bile salts [102].

Interest in the effects of free bile acids derives mainly from the quite recent discovery that stagnation of intestinal contents results in the multiplication of anaerobic bacteria which actively split conjugated bile salts [151, 158] and by the consistent finding of free bile acids in the intestinal lumen of patients with malabsorption and high bacterial counts in the upper small intestine [643, 227]. Some workers believe it is not the presence of free bile acids but the low level of conjugated bile salts that is the cause of the steatorrhoea [645] but the question has not been finally settled.

There is also uncertainty about the significance of a very insoluble bile salt, lithocholate, which in 1961 was shown by Hellström and Sjövall to arise from bacterial reduction of the primary bile salt chenodeoxy-cholate. There has been intense interest in lithocholate since Holsti [317] found that feeding it to rabbits produced cirrhosis of the liver. Other reports have confirmed the extreme hepato-toxicity of this agent, and have shown that it can also induce gallstone formation [502, 95]. Furthermore, lithocholate produces fever, systemic symptoms, and local necrosis when injected intramuscularly in minute quantities [501]. Inevitably there has been much speculation on possible pathogenic roles of lithocholate in man but to date the evidence is still scanty. The three diseases considered most likely to be lithocholate-related are cirrhosis of the liver [88], intrahepatic cholestasis [557] and cholelithiasis [602] especially when there is excessive exposure of bile salts to intestinal bacteria [285]. An interesting new development is the discovery that the liver 'detoxicates' lithocholate by adding a sulphate group [499]. Sulphation may be protective by reducing the toxicity of lithocholate [499] and by limiting its intestinal absorption. [413].

THE CLINICAL SIGNIFICANCE OF BILE SALTS

The age-old conviction that bile is important in health and disease has been vindicated in the last few years by many discoveries relating bile salts to clinical problems. The case of the stagnant loop syndrome has already been mentioned. Two other conditions have been identified in which lack of bile salts in the upper small bowel contributes to steatorrhoea. These are resection or disease of the terminal ileum [270, 673], where there is such severe malabsorption of bile salts [622, 426] that one can speak of a break-down of the enterohepatic circulation [17, 280], and non-alcoholic cirrhosis of the liver [20], where there is either impaired synthesis or secretion of bile salts.

A development of much practical importance has been the manufacture of an anion-exchange resin, cholestyramine, which has potent bile salt binding properties. Oral treatment with this agent is sometimes dramatically successful in stopping the watery diarrhoea of patients with bile salt catharsis due to ileal dysfunction [541, 312]. Cholestyramine has also been described as 'a boon to some who itch' [556], because of the relief it brings to patients whose pruritus is due to incomplete cholestasis [87, 677]. A further use of cholestyramine is the lowering of serum cholesterol levels, for which it is sometimes the drug of choice [183].

Bile salts have been at the centre of recent developments in our understanding of the pathogenesis of cholesterol gallstones. Although it was suggested over a hundred years ago that the essence of the problem was a lack of bile salts relative to cholesterol in the bile [385], it is only in the last few years that the physicochemical situation in bile has been clarified [345, 314, 62]. The work of Admirand and Small [4] implies that the defect in stone-forming bile is failure to provide enough micelles for the carriage of cholesterol, while the recent report of Vlahcevic et al. [679] suggests that this failure is due to a too small circulating pool of bile salts. This may have therapeutic as well as theoretical implications, since feeding bile salts has been shown to turn 'bad' bile into 'good' bile [656]. However, it must be stated that at present there are no clear indications for the use of bile salts in clinical practice.

2 Terminology, Basic Chemistry and Distribution

The proper nomenclature of bile salts is so complex as to be virtually incomprehensible to all except steroid chemists. Fortunately, a detailed knowledge of this nomenclature is unnecessary for non-chemists, who can cling gratefully to what the chemists are pleased to call 'trivial names'. The advantage of the trivial name may be illustrated by the fact that the most familiar bile acid, taurocholic acid, is properly named 3α, 7α, 12α-trihydroxy-5β-cholan-24-oyltaurine. Those wishing to master the intricacies of steroid nomenclature are referred to *Biochemistry* **8**, 2227 (1969).

It is however essential to know something of the terminology and chemistry of bile salts to understand their metabolism and their role in health and disease.

BILE ACID VERSUS BILE SALT

The terms bile acid and bile salt are commonly used interchangeably. Strictly speaking, the choice of expression should depend on the state of ionisation, so that the unionised material is the acid and the ionised form is the salt. To confuse matters, there is a tradition of applying the term bile acid to the free or unconjugated material and the term bile salt to the conjugated form. Since there is no general agreement on these points I have continued in this work the practice of using bile acid and bile salt synonymously. It may, however, be pointed out that in normal man bile salts are for most of the time both conjugated and ionised.

BILE SALTS AS STEROIDS

Bile salts share with the other steroids such as sex hormones and adrenal cortical hormones the four-ring nucleus, perhydrocyclopentano-phenanthrene. The four rings are identified by the letters A to D.

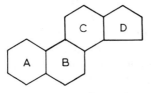

Fig. 2.1. Perhydrocyclopentanophenanthrene, the steroid nucleus.

Bile salts differ most obviously from steroid hormones in having a 5-carbon chain attached to ring D. The basic or prototype bile acid is cholanic acid:

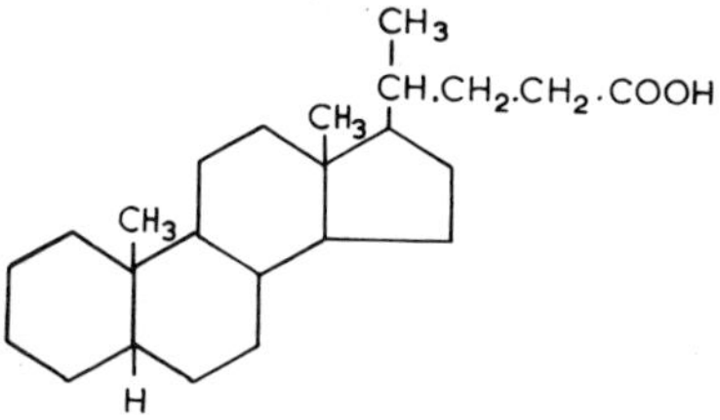

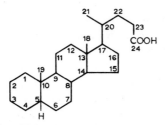

Fig. 2.2. Cholanic acid (5β-cholanoic acid).

Besides the side chain two methyl groups have been added to the nucleus, giving a total complement of 24 carbon atoms. It is important to know how these carbon atoms are numbered. This is shown with the next formula (Fig. 2.3), which is otherwise drawn in the conventional shorthand of bile salt chemistry. The most important carbon atoms from the point of view of substitution and reaction are 3, 7, 12 and 24.

Fig. 2.3. Cholanic acid showing the numbering of the carbon atoms.

SOME CONSIDERATIONS OF SHAPE

In reality the bile salt molecule is not of course flat like its formula. Substituent groups on the nucleus are angled away from the ring structure. Angulation to the front (i.e. towards the observer) is called β-orientation and is indicated by a solid line. Angulation backwards (i.e. away from the observer) is called α-orientation and is indicated by a dashed line. In the formulae of cholanic acid above, both the methyl groups are shown as being in the β orientation. This is the universal situation with bile acids of all species. In the case of the hydrogen atom at C-5 the orientation is variable. In man and most other species it is β-orientated, as shown in the formula of cholanic acid (which is often called 5β-cholanoic acid). Since it is on the same side of the nucleus as the methyl group at C-10, the 5β hydrogen atom is said to be in the *cis* position (Latin *cis* on this side). An alternative expression of the same situation is to say that rings A and B have a *cis* juncture, or briefly that we have an A/B *cis* molecule. The opposite of this normal configuration is the 5α or A/B *trans* molecule, which is called the allo configuration (Fig. 2.4).

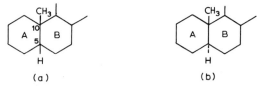

Fig. 2.4. Steric variations at the A/B ring juncture. (a) A/B *cis* or normal configuration (5β hydrogen). (b) A/B *trans* or allo configuration (5α hydrogen).

An example of an allo bile acid is allocholic acid (5α-cholanoic acid) which is an important bile acid in lizards. It has also proved useful in experiments on gallstone formation (see Chapter 12).

The conventional formulae used so far obscure the fact that with ordinary bile acids the molecule is kinked or L-shaped. This can be best shown by means of a perspective formula (Fig. 2.5). The kink is at the A/B ring junction and is determined by the β position of the 5 hydrogen atom. Therefore the L-shape is characteristic of all A/B *cis* or 'normal' bile acids. The L-shape is acquired during the biosynthesis of bile acids from cholesterol. It has been suggested that the kink makes the bile acid molecule resistant to close packing, and therefore to crystallisation, clearly a desirable property in a solubilising agent.

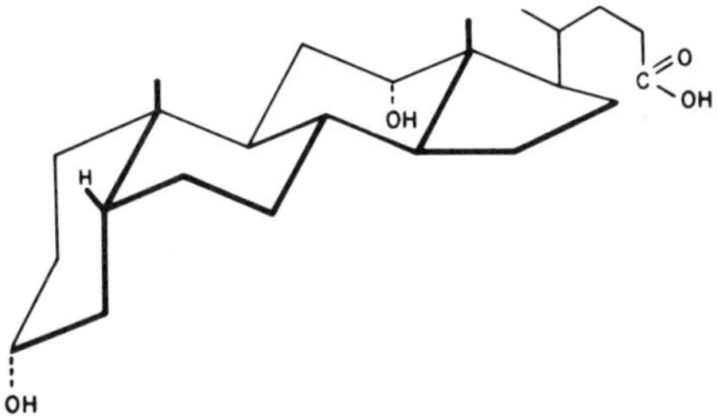

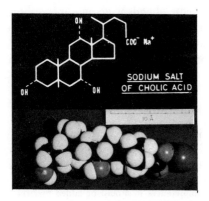

Fig. 2.5. Perspective formula of deoxycholic acid (from Hofmann [304]).

The same α/β terminology is applied to hydroxyl groups. Almost all the important natural bile acids have hydroxyl groups substituted for hydrogen atoms at one or more of four positions, C-3, C-6, C-7 and C-12. In man the major bile acids all have α hydroxyl groups, which means that the hydroxyl groups are on the opposite side of the molecule to the methyl groups. The important implication of this is that one side of the molecule is entirely hydrocarbon and inert while the other side bears groups which are physicochemically active. This point is best illustrated by a model of a bile salt molecule (Fig. 2.6) which also shows that the carboxyl group on the side chain is on the same side as the hydroxyl groups.

Fig. 2.6. A molecular model of cholic acid.

BILE ACIDS OF MAN

Human bile contains three main bile acids, cholic, chenodeoxycholic and deoxycholic, with minute amounts of a fourth, lithocholic.* All four acids have an α-hydroxyl group in the C-3 position. A 7α-OH group is present in cholic and chenodeoxycholic acids and a 12α-OH group in cholic and deoxycholic acids. Therefore we have one tri-hydroxy (cholic), two di-hydroxy (chenodeoxycholic and deoxycholic) and one mono-hydroxy bile acid (Fig. 2.7).

PRIMARY AND SECONDARY BILE ACIDS

Figure 2.7 classifies cholic and chenodeoxycholic as primary, deoxycholic and lithocholic as secondary bile acids. Primary bile acids are those which are synthesised in the liver cell. They would be the only bile acids in bile if there were no enterohepatic circulation. However about 20 per cent of human biliary bile acids are secondary. Secondary bile acids are derived from primary bile acids by the action of bacteria in the intestine. These bacteria have a predilection for removing the 7α-hydroxyl group and the results of their attentions are the conversion of cholic to deoxycholic acid, and of chenodeoxycholic to lithocholic acid. Other bacterial alterations take place to some extent (as discussed in Chapter 6), so that there are many other secondary bile acids in the faeces. However none except deoxycholic and lithocholic are absorbed and recirculated to any significant extent, so that for practical purposes these are the only two secondary bile acids in bile. Of the two, deoxycholic is far more abundant because it is reabsorbed much better than lithocholic. Lithocholic acid is present in such small amounts that it is often ignored in accounts of the composition of bile. The origin and significance of secondary bile acids are discussed in greater detail in Chapters 6, 9 and 10.

CONJUGATION

Up to this point bile salts have been considered only in their free or unconjugated state. However, when they leave the liver cell and enter the biliary tract bile salts are for practical purposes entirely in the

* For the sake of completeness it should be added that traces of the following have also been identified in human bile—ursodeoxycholic, allocholic, 3α, 7α, 12α-trihydroxy coprostanic and 3α, 7α-dihydroxy coprostanic acids [275, 95].

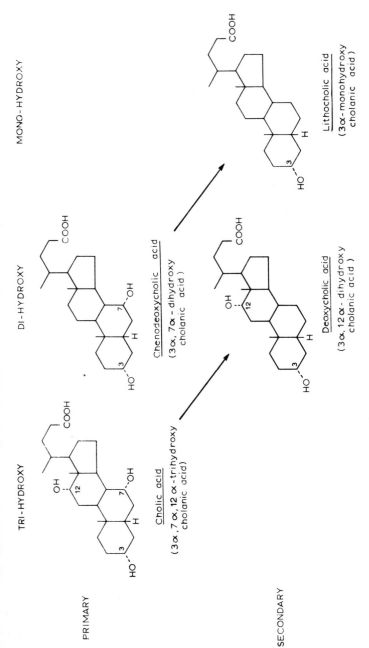

Fig. 2.7. The important circulating bile acids of man, classified (a) by the number of hydroxyl groups on the steroid nucleus and (b) into primary and secondary bile acids.

conjugated form. Conjugation of a bile salt consists of the addition of an amino-acid, glycine or taurine, by peptide (amide) linkage to the carboxyl group of the side chain (Fig. 2.8). This peptide link is unique in its resistance to natural peptidases and to laboratory hydrolysis [467].

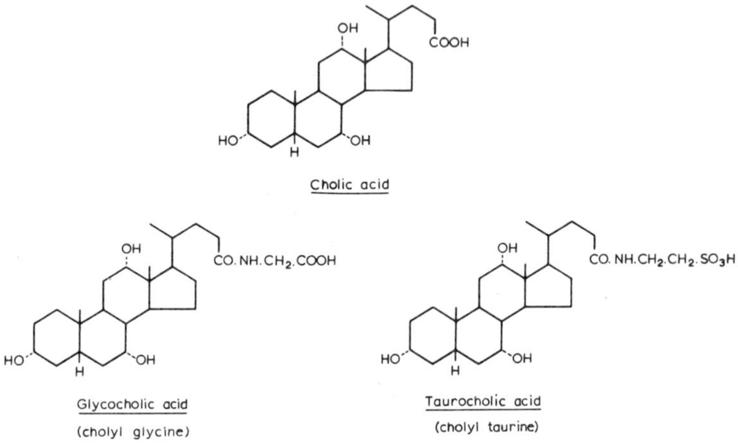

Cholic acid

Glycocholic acid
(cholyl glycine)

Taurocholic acid
(cholyl taurine)

Fig. 2.8. Cholic acid and its two conjugates.

The three main bile acids of man are all conjugated in this way (probably lithocholic acid also, but information is scanty). Therefore the actual bile salts present in human bile, ignoring trace materials, are six in number:

Glycocholate (GC)
Taurocholate (TC)
Glycochenodeoxycholate (GCDC)
Taurochenodeoxycholate (TCDC)
Glycodeoxycholate (GDC)
Taurodeoxycholate (TDC)

The ratio of glycine-conjugated to taurine-conjugated bile salts (G/T ratio) is variable, but in normal subjects it usually lies between 1 and 6 [116, 212, 419, 596] with a mean of 3.2 [596].

THE COMPOSITION OF THE BILE SALT POOL

This is governed by two molar ratios, the G/T ratio and the cholic : chenodeoxycholic : deoxycholic or C : CDC : DC ratio. The latter ratio is also very variable. The normal figures most widely quoted are 1.1 : 1 : 0.6, which are the average results obtained by Sjövall [596] in 21 mostly male Swedish medical students. The average values given recently by Dam *et al.* [116] for 42 mostly female young Danes were 1.26 : 1 : 0.71. In the author's laboratory the average ratios obtained in 19 normal subjects are 1.4 : 1 : 0.9 [454], while values obtained in Japan were 1.39 : 1 : 0.35 [336].

A different and possibly more useful way of expressing the relative proportions of the three (unconjugated) bile acids is as percentages of the total. Thus Sjövall's C : CDC : DC of 1.1 : 1 : 0.6 becomes C 41 per cent, CDC 37 per cent, DC 22 per cent.

A third way suggested by Hofmann is to plot the percentages on triangular co-ordinates, so that each set of data is represented by a single point (see p. 39).

With the spread of gas liquid chromatography, data are appearing on the proportion of lithocholate in the bile salt pool. In American male hospital controls, lithocholate comprises about 2 per cent of the pool [684].

An expression sometimes used to describe bile-salt composition is the tri-hydroxy/di-hydroxy ratio (tri-OH/di-OH or T/D ratio). This arose from the technical difficulty of separating the two di-hydroxy bile salts from each other by methods other than gas liquid chromatography. It is obviously less informative than the C : CDC : DC ratio.

There is no quick and easy way of combining the G/T and C : CDC : DC ratios to express the relative proportions of all six main bile salts in human bile. Perhaps the most graphic method is a circular diagram as in Fig. 2.9.

BILE SALTS IN THE FOETUS AND CHILD [514, 173]

The human foetus conjugates almost exclusively with taurine. After birth glycine conjugates increase gradually until the adult G/T ratio is reached after a few months. Deoxycholate is absent in infants under a year old and the T/D ratio is high for several years.

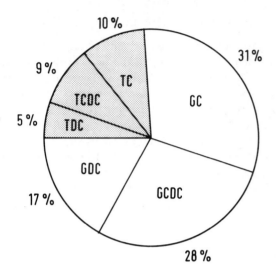

Fig. 2.9. Relative proportions of the six main bile salts in human bile (average values, based on Sjövall [596]).

BILE ACIDS IN OTHER SPECIES

This subject has been extensively studied and fully discussed by Haslewood [275]. He has been able to show that the chemical structure of the bile acids in a given vertebrate species reflects the place of that species in the evolutionary tree [274]. The most primitive vertebrates (e.g. coelacanths, sharks) have 27-carbon bile alcohol sulphates instead of bile acids. Other fish and amphibians have a mixture of bile alcohols and bile acids. Reptiles tend to have primitive bile acids such as allocholic acid and hydroxylated coprostanic acid (a 27-carbon molecule). Birds and mammals both have mostly the 24-carbon cholic and chenodeoxycholic acids, which are presumably the most recently evolved bile acids. With respect to conjugation, taurine is the sole amino acid in all species except mammals. Amongst mammals, carnivores tend to be taurine conjugaters of mainly cholic acid while herbivores and omnivores have a considerable amount of di-hydroxy bile acids and often of glycine conjugates [275].

GENERAL CHEMICAL PROPERTIES OF BILE SALTS

Bile salts are colourless, crystalline solids with an intensely bitter taste. Their solubility in water varies greatly. The free acids are rather poorly soluble but the sodium salts are freely soluble. Conjugation, especially with taurine, greatly increases water solubility. Otherwise solubility is directly proportional to the number of hydroxyl groups on the nucleus. The monohydroxy bile salt, lithocholate, is highly insoluble and curiously its conjugates are less soluble than the free salt [606]. All acids and salts are quite soluble in alcohol.

For detailed accounts of the chemistry of bile salts see references 188, 275, 614, 672 and especially 467a.

3 Physicochemical Properties of Bile Salts in Relation to their Structure and Function. Natural Detergents

Of all the recent advances in our understanding of bile salts, perhaps the most fascinating has been the discovery of how their chemical structure fits them for their role as natural detergents. Much of our knowledge in this field derives from the work of A. F. Hofmann and D. M. Small and their colleagues, and they have published several masterly reviews [97, 304, 307, 309, 314, 603, 604], which are essential reading for anyone wishing to study the subject in depth.

To the clinician this aspect of bile salts is important because loss of detergency underlies several malabsorption syndromes [305], because gallstones probably result from bile being a substandard detergent [603] and because detergent in the wrong part of the body is likely to be harmful [279].

THE CLASSIFICATION OF DETERGENTS

Detergents are substances with the power to disperse water-insoluble lipids into clear aqueous solution. They are sometimes classified according to the electrical charge on the molecule into anionic (negatively charged), cationic (positively charged) and non-ionic or better zwitterionic. The most familiar detergent, household soap, consists of the sodium and potassium salts of long-chain fatty acids. These fatty acids, like bile acids, tend to dissociate or ionise, leaving a negatively charged carboxyl radical:

$$R-COOH \rightleftharpoons R-COO^- + H^+$$

Therefore fatty acid soaps and bile salts are anionic detergents.

A more important classification is into aliphatic or paraffin chain detergents, which are by far the commonest, and a small group of aromatic detergents of which the only important member is the bile salts [97].

THE ESSENTIAL FEATURES OF DETERGENTS

These may be summarised as follows:
(1) They are freely soluble in water.
(2) They are surface-active, that is they lower surface tension at an air-water or oil-water interface.
(3) They form polymolecular aggregates or micelles in water; this is their unique distinguishing feature.

These characteristics are all explained by the structure of the detergent molecule. This has two parts with completely different properties. One part is water-soluble or hydrophilic, the other is water-insoluble or hydrophobic. The water-insoluble part is hydrocarbon, and so inert and fat-soluble. The water-soluble part is called polar because, like a magnet seeking the pole, it is attracted towards water. Strong polarity derives from chemical groups which ionise, such as carboxyl, sulphate and phosphate. Weak polar groups are alcohol (hydroxyl), aldehyde and amine.

Any compound having this dual nature is called an amphiphile (Greek = loving both), or amphipath (feeling both). For the amphiphile to be water-soluble the polar part of the molecule must be strong enough to outweigh the water-repellent bulk of the non-polar part. A soluble amphiphile is in fact the correct definition of a detergent. An older but equivalent term is association colloid.

ORDINARY OR ALIPHATIC DETERGENTS

These will be considered first because their simple structure makes them easier to understand than bile salts. There are important differences between the two groups, but the general principles involved are the same. Examples of aliphatic detergents are fatty acid soaps, household detergents, industrial detergents and lysolecithin [97].

A typical aliphatic detergent is sodium lauryl sulphate. This is the sodium salt of a 12-carbon saturated fatty acid which bears a strongly charged sulphate group:

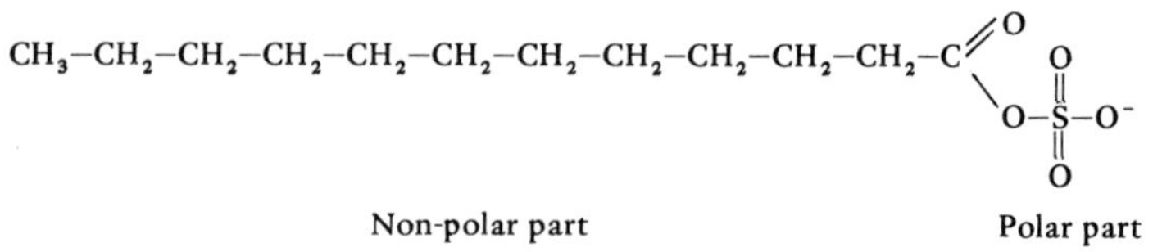

$$CH_3-CH_2-CH_2-CH_2-CH_2-CH_2-CH_2-CH_2-CH_2-CH_2-CH_2-C \overset{\displaystyle O}{\underset{\displaystyle O-\overset{\displaystyle O}{\underset{\displaystyle O}{S}}-O^-}{}}$$

Non-polar part   Polar part

A glance at this formula shows that it divides naturally into two parts, a non-polar paraffin chain and a polar (negatively charged) end-grouping. As a convenient shorthand this type of molecule is drawn like a tadpole, with a polar head and a wavy because flexible tail. (Fig. 3.1).

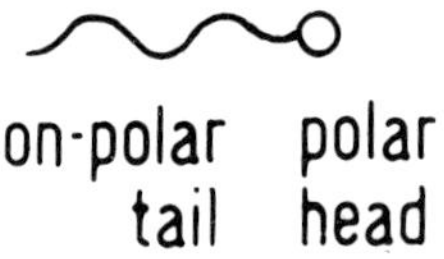

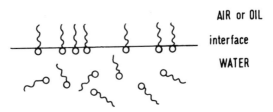

non-polar   polar
   tail   head

Fig. 3.1. A stylised aliphatic detergent molecule.*

This shorthand formula can now be used to demonstrate the three essential features of a detergent as listed above.

(1) It is soluble in water, in spite of its large non-polar (fatty) tail, because the highly charged head causes neighbouring molecules to repel each other.

(2) It lowers surface tension because its molecules tend to line up at an air-water or oil-water interface, with the polar parts projecting downwards into the water (Fig. 3.2).

AIR or OIL

interface

WATER

Fig. 3.2. Molecules of a soluble amphiphile (aliphatic detergent) lining up at an interface.

(3) It forms polymolecular aggregates or micelles because of mutual attraction between the hydrophobic tails. These join together spontaneously to form a sub-microscopic particle with a

* Throughout this chapter an open circle (○) implies a charged polar group, a closed circle (●) a less polar hydroxyl or ester group.

hydrocarbon (oily) centre, round which the hydrophilic heads form a water-soluble shell. Since the polar groups project into the aqueous phase the detergent has neatly solved the problem of satisfying both sides of its nature (Fig. 3.3).

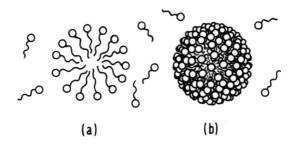

(a) **(b)**

Fig. 3.3. Two aliphatic detergent micelles, (a) in diagrammatic cross-section, and (b) in outside perspective. (The micelle is shown here as being spherical, but it may also be cylindrical.)

For a detergent in solution to form micelles there must of course be enough molecules available. In other words there is a minimum concentration at which micelles start to form. This is called the *critical micellar concentration* or CMC. There is also a critical micellar temperature or CMT, sometimes incorrectly called the Krafft point [97], below which micelles will not form. For lauryl sulphate the CMT is $15\text{-}18^\circ$ C but for the common conjugated bile salts it is well below 0° C and therefore of no physiological significance. Micelles are surrounded by unassociated detergent molecules (monomers) in free solution, and it is believed that molecules exchange rapidly and continuously between the micellar phase and monomer or bulk phase. This led Hofmann to coin the graphic phrase 'flickering clusters'. As the concentration of a detergent is raised above the CMC there is an increase in the number of micelles but not in their size. The concentration of monomers remains constant. This has the important implication that a micellar solution may be very concentrated yet exert an 'anomalously' low osmotic pressure, since osmotic pressure depends on the number of particles present, not on the number of molecules. The relevance to bile in the gallbladder is apparent.

Micellar solutions are optically clear and translucent. This is because micelles are too small to scatter light, their diameter being in the range of 30-100 Angstroms. They are much smaller then emulsion particles (2,000-50,000 Å) which of course do scatter light. Micellar solutions differ further from emulsions in that they are completely stable.

THE DIFFERENCES BETWEEN ALIPHATIC DETERGENTS AND BILE SALTS

There is an obvious difference in shape between a bile salt molecule and an aliphatic detergent molecule. The latter has a long flexible hydrophobic tail and a compact polar head (Fig. 3.1). A bile salt molecule has a rigid discoid hydrocarbon body and a fairly short side-chain ending in a highly polar ionic group; the presence of two or three hydroxyl groups on one side of the body makes this side hydrophilic, while the other side remains hydrophobic (Fig. 2.6). Therefore, at an air-water or oil-water interface the bile salt molecule positions itself tangentially rather than on its head (Fig. 3.4). A further difference is in the organisation of the micelle. In a bile salt micelle the molecules are arranged back to hydrophobic back, as shown in Fig. 3.4.

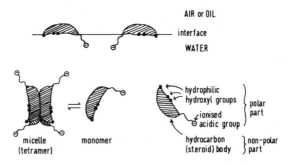

Fig. 3.4. Bile salt molecules lying tangentially at an interface and in solution as monomer and micelle.

In this example, the micelle contains only four bile salt molecules. In general bile salt micelles are much smaller than those of aliphatic detergents, the number of molecules per micelle, or aggregation number, being 4 to 6 for cholate and its conjugates, about 12 for chenodeoxycholate and deoxycholate, and about 18 for their conjugates [314]. The micelles formed by a mixture of conjugated bile salts contain about 10 to 12 molecules under physiological conditions

of pH, temperature and counterion concentration [96] .* For aliphatic
detergents the aggregation number is usually 50-100 [314] .
Experimentally, the size of the bile salt micelle has been shown to be
dependent on the pH, temperature, and sodium concentration of the
solution, but not on the concentration of the bile salt itself [97] .
Under certain circumstances, di-hydroxy bile salts can form quite large
micelles, with an aggregation number of over 60. These larger particles
are probably composed of clusters of micelles hydrogen-bonded
through their hydroxyl groups [97] .

HOW DETERGENTS DISSOLVE LIPIDS;
MICELLAR SOLUBILISATION

When a lipid dissolves in a detergent solution its molecules are
dispersed into the detergent micelles. The simplest form of micellar
solubilisation is that in which a completely non-polar lipid, that is a
hydrocarbon, is taken up into the oily interior of an aliphatic detergent
micelle (Fig. 3.5). This is not an efficient way of dissolving lipid since

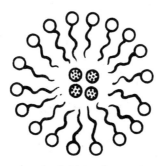

Fig. 3.5. How a non-polar lipid is taken up into a micelle by an
aliphatic detergent.

on average four or five detergent molecules are required to solubilise
one molecule of lipid. Bile salts, in fact are virtually incapable of
dissolving non-polar lipids. This, however is of no consequence since
such lipids are non-physiological.

All lipids of physiological interest are to some extent polar, and are
therefore amphiphiles. The insoluble ones, that is those which require

* Physiologically, however, pure bile salt micelles are not to be found except
perhaps in the lumen of the ileum after meals.

micellar solubilisation, are divided into two classes according to whether or not they interact with water by 'swelling' (see below). These, with their regrettably cumbersome names, are:

(1) Insoluble non-swelling amphiphiles [97]. Examples are long chain fatty acids (unionised), diglycerides, triglycerides, cholesterol and fat-soluble vitamins. These lipids have a polar group which is strong enough to make the molecules orientate themselves at air-water or oil-water interfaces, but is too weak to overcome the mutual attraction between the large hydrocarbon moieties. Consequently when mixed with water these lipids remain totally separate as an oil phase.

(2) Insoluble swelling amphiphiles [97]. Examples are phospholipids (such as lecithin), monoglycerides and some ionised long chain fatty acids. These lipids have a polar group which is still not quite large enough to confer aqueous solubility but which does permit a certain interaction with water, namely 'swelling'. Layers of water molecules interpose themselves between layers of lipid in a curiously organised way, which both expands and imparts flexibility to the lipid (Fig. 3.6). The result is cylindrical or lamellar aggregates which are known as liquid crystals,

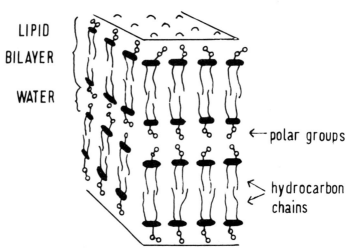

Fig. 3.6. The interaction between water and an insoluble SWELLING amphiphile (lecithin) to form a liquid crystalline phase, in this case a lamellar one.

because they form a phase that is physically liquid but has crystalline features on X-ray analysis. If much water is present the liquid crystals separate out and can be seen under the polarising microscope as impressive structures called myelin figures because they were first seen in an extract of myelin (Fig. 3.7). To the naked eye the 'solution' is turbid and viscous.

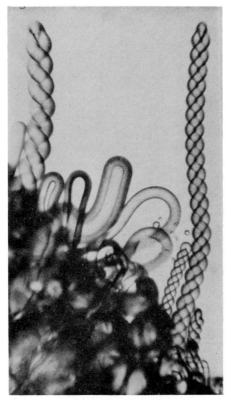

Fig. 3.7. Myelin figures (from Hofmann [307]).

Aliphatic detergents seem to solubilise the two classes of insoluble polar lipids in essentially the same way [97] (Fig. 3.8).

The possession of a polar head allows the insoluble lipid molecule to interdigitate between the detergent molecules. This is a more efficient form of solubilisation than that of a non-polar lipid (Fig. 3.5) since only about two molecules of detergent are required for each molecule

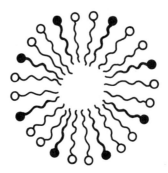

Fig. 3.8. How an insoluble polar liquid is taken up into an aliphatic detergent micelle. An expanded micelle.

of polar lipid [97]. However the main interest of this process is in the fact that the expanded micelle can now take considerably more non-polar lipid into its oily interior. This can be seen by comparing Fig. 3.9 with Fig. 3.5. This process occurs whenever greasy hands are washed with soap and water. The ionised soap molecules act as detergent or soluble amphiphile while the unionised soap molecules (that is fatty acid) act as the polar lipid which expands the micelle. The result is an efficient system for solubilising non-polar lipid, in other words for removing grease and associated dirt from the hands. As a general rule any effective detergent solution contains expanded micelles made up of soluble amphiphile and polar lipid.

In the case of *bile salts* there is an extraordinary difference in the efficiency with which swelling and non-swelling insoluble amphiphiles are solubilised. There are several non-swelling amphiphiles which are

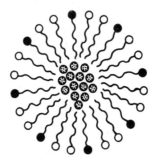

Fig. 3.9. An expanded micelle of aliphatic detergent and polar lipid which has taken up non-polar lipid into its interior.

physiologically important and which have to be solubilised in the bile or the intestinal lumen, for example long chain fatty acids, cholesterol and the fat-soluble vitamins. Of these only the fatty acids can be solubilised at all well, probably in the fashion depicted in Fig. 3.10, but the best that can be achieved is a molar ratio of fatty acid to bile salt (saturation ratio) of under 0.2 [97] *. Cholesterol and vitamin D are

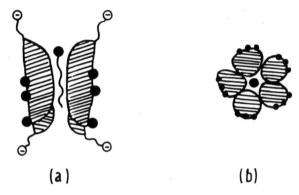

(a)   **(b)**

Fig. 3.10. A bile salt micelle containing a fatty acid molecule (a non-swelling insoluble polar lipid), (a) in longitudinal section, and (b) in cross section.

dissolved even less efficiently, between 19 (glycodeoxycholate) and 62 (taurocholate) molecules of bile salt being required to dissolve one molecule of cholesterol [286], and the precise mechanism involved is unknown [97]. At first sight this suggests that bile salts are less efficient than artificial detergents. However, in life bile salts are never called on to dissolve lipids without the assistance of a swelling amphiphile, so that in fact the wisdom of nature is unshaken.

It is with the swelling polar lipids that the superb efficiency of bile salts is evident. For example, one mole of bile salts can solubilise two moles of lecithin. This feat is probably achieved by a sleeve of bile salts encircling a segment of a liquid crystalline cylinder, that is a double layer of lecithin molecules (the lipid bilayer of Fig. 3.6), and chopping it off into a drum or disc-shaped structure bristling with polar groups

* The saturation ratio rises as the chain length of the fatty acid is decreased so that medium chain fatty acids (with 7 to 10 carbon atoms) have the remarkably high ratio of 3.0 [97]. This has little physiological significance but helps to explain the ready absorption of medium chain triglycerides given therapeutically in cases of bile salt deficiency.

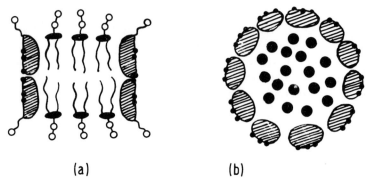

(a)   (b)

Fig. 3.11. A mixed micelle of bile salt and swelling polar lipid (here phospholipid), (a) in longitudinal, (b) in cross section.

(Fig. 3.11). This process is of extreme physiological importance as it is the means by which lecithin is held in solution in bile and by which monoglycerides and some fatty acids are solubilised in the intestine during digestion. The cohesive forces in this micelle are hydrophobic bonds linking the backs of the bile salt molecules with the hydrocarbon chains of the phospholipid or monoglyceride molecules. Incorporation of a swelling amphiphile greatly increases the size of a bile salt micelle and its molecular weight may rise by a factor of 45. At the same time the critical micellar concentration of the bile salt falls from, say, 3 mM to 0.2 mM [97].* Clearly this implies a highly economical use of the body's natural detergent, which at this point is four or five times more efficient than an aliphatic detergent [307].

An important bonus from this process is that the expanded micelle has a much enhanced capacity for solubilising a non-swelling insoluble amphiphile, such as cholesterol and unionised fatty acid. This is superficially similar to the enhanced ability of an aliphatic detergent micelle to dissolve non-polar lipid when it is expanded by polar lipid. However, with a bile salt micelle additional lipid is not buried in the centre of the particle but is sandwiched between the molecules of swelling amphiphile as shown in Fig. 3.12. Three-component micelles of

* The CMC of bile salts is less sharply defined than that of aliphatic detergents. It is lower with dihydroxy bile salts than trihydroxy ones. With a mixture, the CMC lies nearer that of the dihydroxy bile salts. An equimolar mixture of taurine-conjugated di- and tri-hydroxy bile salts has a CMC of 1.6 mM (in 0.15 M sodium chloride at 37° C). This is close to the estimated CMC of actual bile, namely 0.9 to 2.2 mM with a mean of 1.45 mM [647].

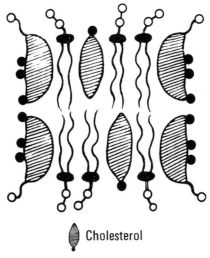

Cholesterol

Fig. 3.12. A bile salt micelle expanded with swelling amphiphile (phospholipid), which has taken up cholesterol, a non-swelling insoluble lipid (modified from Small [603]).

this type are almost certainly present in intestinal content during fat digestion (bile salt—monoglyceride—unionised fatty acid) as well as in bile (bile salt—lecithin—cholesterol). A different model for the digestive micelle, in which the bile salt molecules project outwards from a spherical core [160] seems at present less plausible than the discoid model of Fig. 3.12.

EVIDENCE FOR THE EXISTENCE OF MICELLES *IN VIVO*

Almost all the concepts so far mentioned in this chapter are derived from *in vitro* work with artificial systems. The evidence that bile salt-based micelles actually occur *in vivo* may be summarised as follows:

(a) When bile is subjected to ultracentrifugation or to electrophoresis its behaviour shows that it contains a macromolecular complex in which is found most of the cholesterol, lecithin and bile salts [67, 345]. On dilution or gel filtration this complex is destroyed.

(b) Ultracentrifugation of intestinal content aspirated during digestion reveals a water-clear phase rich in bile salts, monoglycerides and fatty acids [309, 310].

(c) When the concentration of serially diluted bile is plotted against its surface tension, a curve is obtained which shows inflections consistent with the formation of micelles [647].

(d) The osmotic activity of bile is less than expected from its concentration of solutes. Also the activity coefficients of sodium and potassium are reduced, presumably through binding of cations to the surfaces of the negatively charged micelles [446].

(e) Electron microscopy of bile has revealed cigar-shaped particles about 100 Å long [326] (Fig. 3.13). Their striped appearance

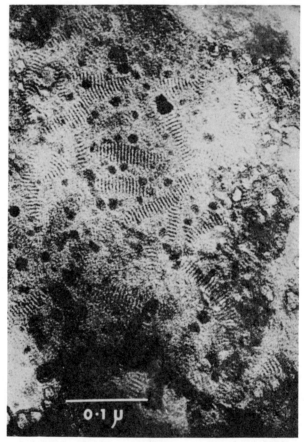

Fig. 3.13. (a) Striped cigar-shaped assemblies in human bile (×280,000). (b) The same—in artificial bile (from Howell *et al.*) , [326].

has been interpreted as representing a structure in which disc-shaped micelles are stacked together but separated by layers of electron-dense water (Fig. 3.14).

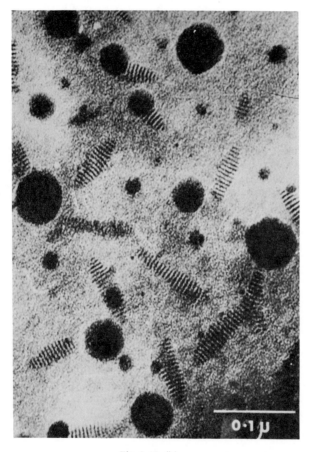

Fig. 3.13. (b)

(f) Artificial mixtures of bile salts, lecithin and cholesterol have physicochemical [314] and electron microscopic [326] properties similar to those of bile.

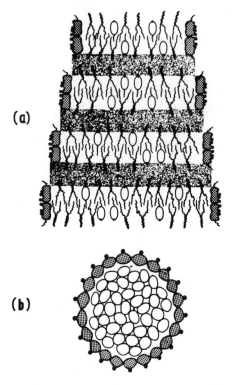

Fig. 3.14. Possible organisation of one end of a cigar-shaped assembly, formed by the association of disc-shaped mixed micelles of bile salts, phospholipid and cholesterol, with intercalated layers of water (from Howell *et al.* [326]).

QUANTITATIVE ASPECTS OF THE INTERACTION
OF BILE SALTS WITH OTHER LIPIDS:
THE USE OF PHASE DIAGRAMS

As stated earlier, in life bile salt solutions generally contain both kinds of insoluble polar lipid, swelling and non-swelling. The optimal physical state of such a three-component mixture is a micellar solution, but clearly this will be achieved only if the relative proportions of the components are within certain limits. Outside these limits one or both lipids will come out of solution as crystals, liquid crystals or oil droplets depending on their relative proportions. An elegant and convenient way of expressing these proportions and also the predicted physical states of mixtures is to construct phase diagrams. These are equilateral triangles each side of which concerns the molar concentration of one component, expressed as a percentage of the total number of moles in the mixture. The composition of any three-component mixture can be plotted as a single point, as shown in Fig. 3.15. Such a figure is

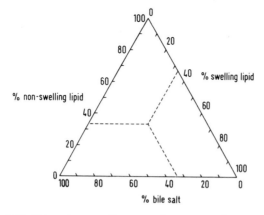

Fig. 3.15. Triangular co-ordinates used to express the composition of a 3-component mixture of bile salt and two insoluble polar lipids, swelling and non-swelling. The point in the middle of the triangle represents a mixture of equal parts (33⅓ per cent) of each component.

converted into a phase diagram by indicating which areas within the triangle (that is, which ranges of relative concentrations) correspond with which observed physical states or phase equilibria. This is done by making up large numbers of mixtures of all possible proportions and observing their physical state by techniques such as microscopy and X-ray diffraction. The amount of water present, that is the total concentration of solids, must be defined for each diagram since it may influence the phase equilibria.*

* If the phase diagram technique is to be used to show in addition the phase variations induced by different water concentrations, it is necessary to construct a three-dimensional model in the shape of a regular tetrahedron (prism). Fortunately this is not necessary in the study of human gallbladder bile, since the variations in water content are usually within the range of 80-95 per cent, in which the phase equilibria do not vary materially [4].

The triple mixture of bile salt, lecithin and cholesterol has been extensively studied in this way by Small and his colleagues [607] and they have shown that, at physiological water content, only mixtures in the lower left hand part of the triangle are fully soluble, presumably as micellar solutions (Fig. 3.16). Outside the micellar zone, mixtures

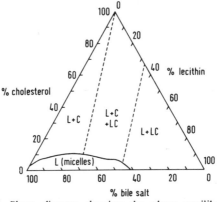

Fig. 3.16. Phase diagram showing the phase equilibria of bile salt–lecithin–cholesterol mixtures at 90 per cent water content and 37°C (modified from Admirand & Small [4]). L = liquid, C = crystals, LC = liquid crystals.

contain crystals of cholesterol, or liquid crystals of lecithin with or without cholesterol. Bile has been found to behave like this model system, presumably because its other components are small in quantity and freely soluble (mainly bilirubin and electrolytes). Consequently it is becoming a popular practice to assess the degree of cholesterol-saturation of bile specimens by plotting their composition using triangular co-ordinates (see Chapter 12).

Rather little is known of the size of the biliary micelles, because it is difficult to use analytical methods which do not or may not alter or destroy the micelles [97]. Estimated molecular weights range from 11,000 [67] to 150,000 [97] but it seems certain that micelles in gallbladder bile are four or five times larger than micelles in the less concentrated hepatic bile [67].

Still less is known of the micelles and phase equilibria of upper small bowel content during digestion. The situation is complex and rapidly changing. However, it is likely that the micelles are composed chiefly of bile salt, monoglyceride and fatty acid and that their general structure is as in Fig. 3.12 [97, 314].

pH, pK_a AND CONJUGATION

Like all weak acids, bile acids are only partly ionised or dissociated at physiological pH values:

$$HA \rightleftharpoons H^+ + A^-$$

The pK_a * of a weak acid is the pH at which half is ionised and half unionised. The pK_a is a useful index of the tendency to ionise and therefore of the strength of a weak acid. The lower the pK_a, the stronger the acid. Further, since ionisation increases solubility in water, the lower the pK_a the more soluble is the acid in solutions of low pH.

With bile acids the pK_a has special significance. Above their CMCs, the free bile acids cholic, chenodeoxycholic and deoxycholic all have a pK_a of about 6, their glycine conjugates about 4.7, and their taurine conjugates about 2.5 (below the CMC, pK_a values are about 1.0 lower [307]). Thus conjugation, especially with taurine, has a notable effect on the physicochemical properties of bile acids. In particular, while the free bile salts are precipitated from solution (in their acid form, HA) at pH 6.5, the glycine conjugates remain in solution to about pH 4.5, while the taurine conjugates are freely soluble even in their fully unionised form [156]. This resistance to acid precipitation constitutes a major difference between taurine and glycine conjugates, and it would seem to confer a clear advantage on taurine conjugation (which also gives immunity to precipitation by calcium and other heavy metals). It is puzzling therefore that mammals, alone among vertebrates, have developed glycine conjugation [314].

The pK_a is also an indicator of the tendency to diffuse across biological membranes, since non-ionic diffusion is much more rapid than ionic diffusion [145] (see Chapter 6). Therefore, conjugation of bile acids has the effect of limiting their 'leakage' out of the biliary tract and out of the upper small intestine. Normally no free bile acids are present in the upper small intestine. If formed through bacterial action they would make no contribution to the detergent function of bile salts since (a) they would probably be precipitated at the jejunal pH of about 6, and (b) they would disappear through passive non-ionic diffusion out of the lumen [298].

---

* The strict definition of pK_a is $-\log K_a$, where K_a is the dissociation constant $[H^+] \times [A^-]/[HA]$.

4 Methodology

A comprehensive discussion of the many techniques that have been used to study bile salts and their metabolism is beyond the scope of this work. The possible experimental approaches are innumerable, ranging from studies in living human subjects or animals, through perfusion of isolated organs and incubation of tissue homogenates or subcellular fractions, down to enzymatic and chemical investigations. The complexity of this field makes a multi-disciplinary team approach most desirable.

The problems that are common to most studies are threefold: extraction of bile salts from complex biological mixtures, separation of the individual bile salts from each other and quantitative estimation of the separated materials.

Many useful facts, references and practical details are to be found in the review of Hofmann *et al.* [313].

EXTRACTION

Bile salts may be extracted from bile, intestinal contents, faeces, blood, urine, and tissues such as liver and intestinal mucosa. The procedure is easiest in bile and fasting intestinal contents, where bile salts are present in high concentration in a relatively simple medium. With the other fluids and tissues very complex methods have been developed. The amount of extraction required depends on which separation technique is to be used subsequently. Bile can be applied directly to a thin-layer silica gel plate but must be extracted several times before gas chromatography.

Details of extraction procedures are to be found in papers describing the different separation and assay techniques. Ethanol (95 per cent or more) and methanol are the most generally useful extractants for conjugated bile salts. When used in five-fold excess they precipitate proteins including mucus and much of the bile pigment. The neutral fats and sterols can be largely extracted with petrol ether or ether-heptane (1 : 1, V/V). To extract free bile acids, acidification to pH 2 with concentrated HCl may be followed by extraction with chloroform-methanol 2 : 1.

SEPARATION

The many techniques that can be used to separate individual bile salts were reviewed by Sjövall [597]. He classified them into four groups: adsorption chromatography (column, glass-paper and thin-layer); counter-current distribution; partition chromatography (liquid-liquid column especially reversed phase chromatography, paper, and gas-liquid chromatography); electrophoresis and ion-exchange chromatography.

At present the most popular method is *thin-layer chromatography* using silica gel G or H (Merck). It is simple, rapid, and reasonably sensitive, and can be used for separating conjugated as well as free bile salts. A number of useful solvent systems have been described and these are tabulated in Table 4.1. A disadvantage of thin-layer chromatography is the difficulty of separating the conjugates of deoxycholate from those of chenodeoxycholate, but some success with the glycine conjugates has been claimed by McLeod & Wiggins [419] and by Gregg [239]. Various refinements of the traditional technique have been reported. Thus, Kottke *et al.* [368] washed the silica gel with sulphuric and hydrochloric acids and obtained better separation of deoxycholic and chenodeoxycholic acids, while Stiehl *et al.* [625] further improved the separation by lowering the temperature to 5° C. Panveliwalla *et al.* [503] used plates 50 cm long and three different solvent systems in sequence to obtain maximum separation of free bile acids and glycine conjugates. Multiple developments in the same solvent system were preferred by Bruusgaard [73]. The latter author stressed the importance of using several different solvent systems if complete separation of a complex mixture of bile salts is required. Hamilton [265] used two-dimensional chromatography with two different solvent systems to separate faecal bile acids. Freimuth *et al.* [201] recommend the use of polyamide instead of silica gel to improve the separation of free

TABLE 4.1. *Thin layer chromatographic solvent systems for separating conjugated and free bile acids*

Reference	Conjugated bile salts	Free bile acids
Hofmann (1962)	Iso-amyl acetate : propionic acid : n-propanol : water 4 : 3 : 2 : 1 (does not separate di-hydroxy conjugates, but good for separating GC and GDC-plus-GCDC)	Iso-amyl acetate : di-isopropylether : carbon tetrachloride : n-propanol : benzene : acetic acid 8 : 6 : 4 : 2 : 2 : 1 (also useful for separating taurolithocholate)
Eneroth (1963)		Seventeen different systems, most being composed of varying proportions of 1. Benzene, dioxane and acetic acid, or 2. Cyclohexane, ethyl acetate, acetic acid, or 3. Iso-octane, isopropyl alcohol, acetic acid, or 4. Iso-octane, ethyl acetate, acetic acid (5 : 5 : 1 especially good for separating free bile acids, also LC from GLC)
Gänshirt et al. (1960)	Butanol : acetic acid : water 10 : 1 : 1 (good for separating TC from TDC + TCDC) Toluene : acetic acid : water 10 : 10 : 1 (general purposes)	Toluene : acetic acid : water 5 : 5 : 1 (using upper non-aqueous phase)
Hamilton (1963)		Iso-propyl ether : butanone : acetic acid 100 : 40 : 7 Iso-octane : acetic acid : iso-propyl ether 10 : 6 : 5
Stiehl et al. (1969)		Iso-octane : ethyl acetate : acetic acid 10 : 5 : 2 and 10 : 3 : 2 (for use at 5°C) (separates DC and CDC very well)

TABLE 4.1 *cont.*

Reference	Conjugated bile salts	Free bile acids
Gregg (1966)	Iso-octane : isopropyl ether : acetic acid : iso-propanol 2 : 1 : 1 : 1 (gives good separation of GDC and GCDC in amounts of 20 μg or less) Ethylene dichloride : acetic acid : water 10 : 10 : 1	As for conjugates (first system gives some separation of DC and CDC)
McLeod & Wiggins (1968)	Di-isopropyl ether : acetic acid : 0.5N sulphuric acid 11 : 7 : 2 (separates GDC and GCDC. Whatman SG 41 silica gel used and prepared with 0.5N sulphuric acid)	
Grütte & Gärtner (1969)		Iso-octane : acetic acid : isopropyl ether : isopropyl alcohol 10 : 6 : 5 : 1 (good for separating free di-hydroxy bile acids)
Usui (1963)	Ethyl acetate : acetic acid : methanol 7 : 1 : 2 (no separation of deoxycholates from chenodeoxycholates)	Benzene : acetic acid 8 : 2 (no separation of DC and CDC) (other systems given for methyl esters and keto bile acids)

Abbreviations: GC glycocholate, GDC glycodeoxycholate, GCDC glycochenodeoxycholate, GLC glycolithocholate, TC taurocholate, TDC taurodeoxycholate, TCDC taurochenodeoxycholate, DC deoxycholate, CDC chenodeoxycholate, LC lithocholate.

di-hydroxy bile acids. For detailed accounts of adsorbents, plate preparation, sample application, development techniques, and choice of solvent and detection reagents, the reader is referred to the excellent reviews by Hofmann [303] and by Eneroth [175].

Gas-liquid chromatography (GLC) is a uniquely sensitive and versatile investigative tool and Sjövall [598] has predicted that 'it will become the major technique for the analysis of bile acids on a micro scale'. This prophecy has already been fulfilled in America but not so far in Europe, perhaps because the equipment is expensive and requires skilled attention. It has the great advantage of quantitating at the same time as separating. Its main disadvantage is that it cannot be used for analysing taurine-conjugated bile salts, so that it gives no information on the glycine/taurine conjugation ratio or the extent of deconjugation. Analysis of bile salt mixtures has to be preceded by *hydrolysis*. This is traditionally carried out by heating with sodium or potassium hydroxide under pressure, in an autoclave or steel 'bomb' or sealed glass tube. For example, Swell [635] recommends autoclaving at 15 lb pressure with KOH (final concentration 1.25 N) for three hours. It has been claimed that this type of treatment destroys certain bile acids, and to overcome this Nair & Garcia [465] recommend an enzymatic hydrolysis using the enzyme cholylglycine hydrolase which is derived from clostridial bacteria [467].

Whichever hydrolytic technique is used, the free bile acids must be methylated and preferably converted to the trifluoroacetate derivatives [597] or the trimethylsilyl ether derivatives [422, 246] before being injected into the gas chromatograph.

Identity of retention time with a known standard on gas chromatography has no more significance than identity of distance moved (or more specifically of R_f value) on thin-layer chromatography. For positive identification of an unknown bile acid, GLC should be combined with mass spectrometry. This sophisticated procedure has been described by Sjövall [598]. For an exhaustive account of the technical aspects and applications of gas chromatography of bile acids, the reader is referred to the review by Kuksis [374].

QUANTITATIVE ESTIMATION

Innumerable methods have been published for the measurement of bile salts in biological fluids. Many of these spring from the mid-nineteenth century discovery of Pettenkofer that when bile acids are heated with certain sugars in the presence of concentrated sulphuric acid a purple colour is produced. All these colorimetric reactions have problems of specificity, so it was an important advance when recently an enzymatic reaction was introduced which is specific for bile acids with a 3-hydroxyl group.

At present the most popular methods (apart from GLC) are:

(1) An enzymatic method using β-steroid dehydrogenase.

(2) Sulphuric acid chromogen methods.

(3) Colour reactions for specific bile acids.

ENZYMATIC DETERMINATION

This sensitive and simple technique has in the last few years become used throughout the world. Its principle is as follows: under the influence of the enzyme steroid dehydrogenase, the hydrogen atom of the 3α hydroxyl group from each bile salt molecule is transferred to a NAD molecule and the concentration of the resultant $NADH_2$ is measured spectrophotometrically. The method was originally developed for determining steroid hormones [646] and was adapted for bile salt assay by Iwata and Yamasaki [335]. All naturally occurring bile acids are measured. In practice a crude extract of *Pseudomonas testosteroni* is used as a source of enzyme. The addition of hydrazine hydrate to trap $NADH_2$ ensures a more quantitative relationship between the number of micromoles of bile acid oxidised and the number of micromoles of NAD reduced but it is not absolutely necessary. This method is ideal for measuring the total bile salt content of bile or small bowel aspirate, and details of its use for this purpose are given by Admirand and Small [4] and by Turnberg and Anthony-Mote [668]. The latter workers established the optimal pH, temperature and duration of the reaction as being pH 10, $26°C$ and 40 minutes. At low concentrations there is a slight tendency to over-estimate cholates, and at high concentrations to under-estimate di-hydroxy bile salts. A useful extension of this method is the quantitation of individual bile salt fractions after separation by thin-layer chromatography. The appropriate areas of silica gel are conveniently and efficiently extracted with the pyrophosphate buffer used in the enzymatic reaction [281]. Alternatively the reaction may be carried out with the silica in the tube [73].

Although it was originally described for measuring blood bile acids, the enzymatic method is barely sensitive enough for this purpose. A useful increase in sensitivity has been reported by the use of fluorimetry instead of spectrophotometry to measure the reduced NAD [461].

SULPHURIC ACID CHROMOGEN METHODS [597, 672]

When heated with concentrated or 65 per cent sulphuric acid, most steroids including bile acids form compounds which absorb ultraviolet light and which can therefore be measured with a spectrophotometer. Because this reaction is so non-specific it is necessary first to purify bile acids when working with biological fluids. In the method of Gänshirt *et al.* [211] thin-layer chromatography is followed by scraping the appropriate areas of silica gel straight into the reaction tubes and incubating with 3 ml 65 per cent sulphuric acid at 60° C. Attempts have been made to exploit differences in wavelength peaks to quantitate individual bile acids in mixtures, but the inevitable inaccuracy of such methods limits their usefulness [597]. The sensitivity of the sulphuric acid method can be increased by using fluorimetry [391, 392].

COLOUR REACTIONS FOR SPECIFIC BILE ACIDS

Cholic acids, free and conjugated, can be quickly and accurately measured by the method of Irvin *et al.* [329]. To 1 ml of an aqueous bile salt solution is added 6 ml of 16 N sulphuric acid and 1 ml of a 1 per cent solution of freshly distilled furfuraldehyde. The tubes are heated at 65° C for 13 min and, after cooling, 5 ml glacial acetic acid is added to stabilise the blue colour which develops. Light absorption at 620 mμ is compared with a water blank and standards put through the reaction. There is little interference from other bile acids [393].

Deoxycholic acid can be rapidly measured by the method of Szalkowski & Mader [641], which depends on the red colour produced by reaction with salicylaldehyde in the presence of sulphuric acid. Bruusgaard [73] has shown that the taurine and glycine conjugates give the same absorption as the free acid and has scaled the method down. To the dried bile salt, or to scraped off silica gel containing it, is added 0.6 ml of a solution consisting of 100 μl salicylaldehyde mixed with 3.4 ml 65 per cent sulphuric acid. After heating at 40° C for 15 minutes and standing for five minutes, 4 ml glacial acetic acid is added and the tubes thoroughly stirred. Silica gel is centrifuged down and, exactly 15 minutes after addition of the acetic acid, the absorbance of the supernatant is read at 700 mμ. The value of this method is that it enables conjugated deoxycholates to be measured in the presence of chenodeoxycholates, and with only slight interference. This bypasses the difficulty of separating the two di-hydroxy bile salts by thin-layer chromatography. The method is very reproducible when applied to the combined glycodeoxy- and glycochenodeoxycholate fraction [454].

Chenodeoxycholic acid. The method of Isaksson [331] can only be used on hydrolysed extracts of bile. It is based on the Lieberman-Burchard reaction, so cholesterol must first be completely removed. Chenodeoxycholic acid can be measured indirectly by determining the deoxycholate content of the combined di-hydroxy fraction by the above method and subtracting it from the result of enzymatic assay of the total bile salt content of the same fraction [73].

Lithocholic acid. After hydrolysis and separation from other bile acids, lithocholate can be determined by utilising the deep rose colour which develops when it is dissolved in 3 ml of acetic acid and 2.5 ml of a ferric chloride-sulphuric acid reagent (freshly prepared by adding 1 ml of a 10 per cent solution of ferric chloride in acetic acid to 100 ml sulphuric acid) and measuring the absorbance at 530 mμ [597]. An alternative method involves heating with a 9 : 1 mixture of sulphuric and acetic acids. [92].

ANALYSIS OF SERUM BILE SALTS

The ready availability of blood samples has resulted in a great deal of effort being expended on techniques for analysing the bile salt content of blood. Unfortunately, it is seldom possible to deduce from analyses of blood what is happening in the main arena of bile salt activity, the enterohepatic circulation. Nevertheless, especially in disease of the liver or biliary tract, it is sometimes helpful to analyse the blood. Technically, the main problems are the very low concentrations of bile salt present, and the co-existence of other interfering compounds. Rather complex extraction and concentration procedures are necessary, prior to separation and quantitation. The older methods, based on sulphuric acid chromogens, with or without separation by column chromatography, were too insensitive to give useful data in normal subjects [543, 86]. Gas liquid chromatography is probably the most sensitive method [549], but requires hydrolysis of bile salts so that no information is obtained about the state of conjugation. This disadvantage is absent from a recently described technique using multiple thin-layer chromatographic separations and fluorimetric assay [503]. A comprehensive discussion of serum bile salt estimation has recently been published [88].

ANALYSIS OF FAECAL BILE ACIDS

The faeces contain such a complex mixture of bile acids in various stages of degradation that chemical analysis is forbiddingly difficult. Probably the only accurate analytical method is gas-liquid chromatography [246, 181], preferably combined with mass spectrometry to ensure definite identification of individual bile acids [176]. Measurement of total faecal bile acids is simplified by the use of radioactive labelling but it is still laborious. The isotope derivative method for total faecal bile acids is based on the fact that, after administration of labelled cholesterol, the faecal end products of cholesterol metabolism have specific activities that closely parallel those of the serum cholesterol. The total radioactivity is measured in the extracted bile acid fraction of the stools and this figure is converted into milligrams by dividing into it the serum cholesterol specific activity. This method is discussed further in Chapter 7.

USES OF RADIOACTIVELY LABELLED BILE SALTS

The great advantage of radioactive techniques is the insight they give into the dynamic state of affairs in the living organism. The uses to which they can be put include the following:

(1) Measurement of bile salt pool size and turnover (see Chapter 7).
(2) Assessment of bile salt excretion rates in different states or on different regimes (see Chapter 7).
(3) Analysis of faecal end products [124, 479].
(4) Study of the formation and recirculation of secondary bile salts [214, 282, 480].
(5) Simple, accurate estimation of bile salt levels in the blood [597] or gastric juice [532].

(6) Detection of abnormal bacterial attack on bile salts. This can be done either by detecting unusually rapid deconjugation or dehydroxylation of labelled bile salt in the duodenal aspirate [435, 214] or, more conveniently, by finding excessive excretion of $^{14}CO_2$ in the breath after administering glycine-1-^{14}C labelled glycocholate [203, 313, 545, 581].

5 Hepatic Synthesis and Metabolism of Bile Salts

Bile salts are synthesised in only one organ, the liver. They are broken down in only one organ, the intestine. Damaged bile salts are repaired in the liver. Apart from these three, no other type of bile salt metabolism is known. This chapter is concerned with the production and repair stages, in other words with synthesis, conjugation and reconjugation. Re-hydroxylation will be mentioned briefly because it occurs in species other then man. Breakdown of bile salts is considered in Chapter 6.

HEPATIC SYNTHESIS

The processes involved in synthesis of bile salts from cholesterol have been elucidated by the classical biochemical techniques of feeding labelled precursors to intact animals or adding them to *in vitro* preparations such as liver slices, liver homogenates or subcellular fractions, and identifying the end products. This work has been done mainly in rats, but most of it applies to man. Detailed reviews of this complex subject have been published by Danielsson [120, 121, 125] and Bergström & Danielsson [37].

If the formulae of cholesterol and cholic acid are compared, it can be seen that bile acid synthesis involves changing the cholesterol molecule in five ways: (a) introducing two α-hydroxyl groups, at positions 7 and 12; (b) changing the orientation of the 3-hydroxyl group from β to α; (c) saturating the double bond between C5 and 6; (d) shortening the side chain by three carbon atoms; and (e) oxidising the terminal carbon atom of the side chain to form a carboxylic acid group. Most of the reactions involved in this transformation have been elucidated and the main pathway of cholic acid synthesis can be represented as occurring in nine steps which are shown in Fig. 5.1 This figure also shows that the main pathway for synthesis of chenodeoxycholic acid is identical except for the omission of the 12α-hydroxylation step. Haslewood [275] has made the interesting suggestion that this is an example of enzyme suppression produced through evolutionary selection in vegetarian species.

It should be noted that all the changes affecting the steroid nucleus (steps 1 to 6) are completed before oxidation of the side chain begins. Compound VII represents the dividing line between nuclear and side-chain reactions since it has acquired the nucleus of cholic acid but still has the side chain of cholesterol. Compound IX and its equivalent without the 12α-hydroxyl group are of interest since these two intermediates are found in alligators and crocodiles as the main bile acids. This suggests that they are evolutionarily primitive bile acids which have persisted in reptiles but have been further improved in mammals by side chain shortening. Nevertheless, traces of both these intermediates have been found in human bile [89, 90].

The locations of the enzymes responsible for these reactions are in most cases known [37, 122]. Reactions 1 to 4 occur in the microsomes, reaction 7 in either mitochondria or microsomes, and reaction 9 in the mitochondria. Soluble enzymes are responsible for reactions 5, 6 and 8 and are necessary in reaction 9.

Reaction 1, the 7α-hydroxylation of cholesterol, is of special interest since it is the rate-limiting step in bile acid formation. It is the point at which feedback inhibition on their own synthesis is exerted by bile acids returning to the liver, as shown in experiments with rats [123, 579] and rabbits [457].

The first three steps are common to the formation of both primary bile acids. When reaction 4, the 12α-hydroxylation step, takes place, the liver cell is committed to making cholic acid rather than chenodeoxycholic acid. This step may be of particular clinical importance because, if it is inhibited, cholic acid cannot be formed and cholesterol catabolism is directed towards chenodeoxycholic acid. There is some evidence that this effect is produced by lithocholic acid [441, 466] and by thyroid hormone [37].

An alternative pathway for the synthesis of chenodeoxycholic acid has been proposed by Mitropoulos and Myant, on the basis of *in vitro* work with rat liver [441]. This pathway is illustrated in Fig. 5.2. Its distinctive feature is that it involves oxidation of the cholesterol side chain before the steroid nucleus is hydroxylated and therefore that lithocholic acid is an intermediate product. The existence of such a pathway is supported by the fact that rats and hamsters infused with the first intermediate, 26-hydroxycholesterol, secrete labelled mono-hydroxy bile acid in their bile [685]. The quantitative significance of this pathway is unknown and it has only recently been shown to occur in man.* Nevertheless, it has been speculated that in disease there may be inhibition of the main 'steroid-ring-hydroxylated-first' pathway and, as a consequence, synthesis by the 'side-chain-oxidised-first' pathway of excessive amounts of toxic monohydroxy bile acids [338].

Laboratory studies have shown two alternative pathways for the nuclear stages of cholic acid synthesis, but they are probably of little importance [37].

The hydroxylating enzymes concerned in bile acid synthesis are probably different from those that hydroxylate drugs [169]. *In vitro* they are not induced by phenobarbitone but *in vivo* there is evidence that phenobarbitone enhances bile salt synthesis [530].

CONJUGATION AND RE-CONJUGATION

Synthesis of cholic and chenodeoxycholic acids is followed immediately by conjugation with glycine or taurine. Similarly free bile acids arriving in the portal blood, including deoxycholic acid and presumably lithocholic acid, are rapidly conjugated prior to biliary secretion. This process has been extensively studied in Sweden using homogenates and

---

* It has been shown that 26-hydroxycholesterol is converted to chenodeoxy-cholic acid in patients with bile fistulae [7a].

Fig. 5.1. Main pathways for the synthesis of cholic and chenodeoxycholic acids from cholesterol. (Wih each compound the new chemical group is indicated by larger lettering and heavier lines.)

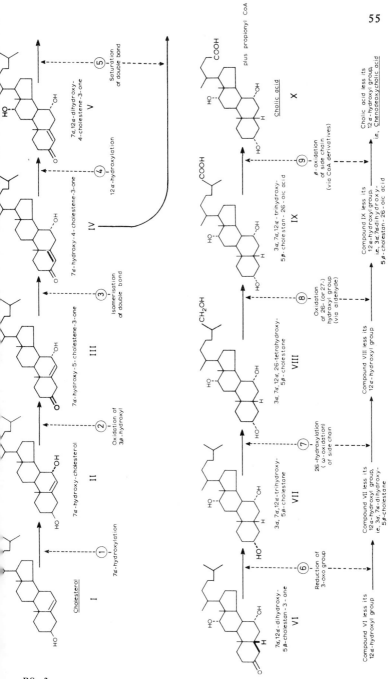

55

BS-3

56

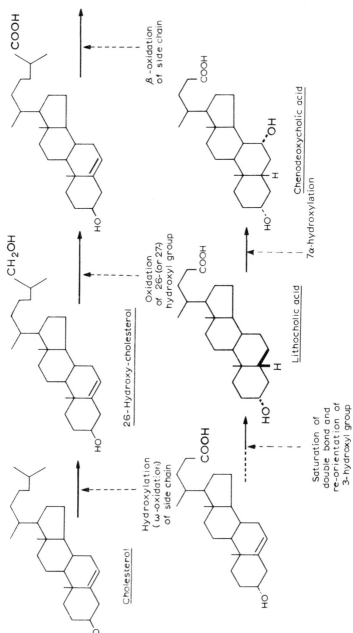

Fig. 5.2. Postulated second pathway for the synthesis of chenodeoxylic acid. (with each compound the new chemical group is indicated by larger lettering and heavier lines.)

subcellular fractions of both rat and human liver [38, 70, 171, 560]. The reaction occurs in two stages. First the bile acid must be 'activated' by formation of the CoA derivative. Then the bile acyl CoA and the amino acid are condensed or conjugated, with the re-formation of CoA, thus:

$$R-CO-S-CoA + H_2N-CH_2-CH_2-SO_3^-$$
Cholyl CoA   Taurate

$$\rightarrow R-CO-NH-CH_2-CH_2-SO_3^- + CoA-SH$$
Cholyl taurate (taurocholate)

The first step is catalysed by the microsomal fraction and requires ATP and Mg^{++}, while the second step requires a lysosomal fraction [560]. Cholic acid added to normal human liver homogenate is conjugated about equally with glycine and taurine but in liver disease glycine conjugation is reduced [170].

The ratio of glycine- to taurine-conjugated bile salts in the bile (G/T ratio) is altered in various disease states and may be of diagnostic value in ileal disorders (see Chapter 10). It is markedly reduced by feeding taurine in doses as small as 1.5 g/day, but is unaffected by large doses of glycine [595, 212]. This suggests that the availability of taurine is an important factor in deciding the level of the G/T ratio.

RE-HYDROXYLATION

In many mammals including man, the liver cannot re-hydroxylate bile acids, such as deoxycholic and lithocholic, which have been dehydroxylated by intestinal organisms prior to absorption. However the rat and the mouse efficiently convert deoxycholate to cholate by 7α-hydroxylation [38] and the rat liver metabolises lithocholate to at least four compounds of greater polarity [657]. This capacity may be protective against the toxic effect of free bile acids. One of the few reactions which seem to be beyond the capacity of the rat is the 12α-hydroxylation of chenodeoxycholate to form cholate. Certain non-mammalian species do however have this capacity [172a].

It is accepted dogma that in man cholate and chenodeoxycholate are metabolically completely distinct from each other.

6 The Enterohepatic Circulation – The Life Cycle of Bile Salts

The enterohepatic circulation or, as it should perhaps be called, the entero-porto-biliary circulation, differs from the other great circulations in that it is a physiological and not an anatomical entity. Though not provided with special vessels it nevertheless keeps within clearly defined anatomical boundaries. Inside these boundaries, bile salts are created, used, moved and metabolised, and from them they escape only to make their last journey out of the body. It is in essence an efficient recycling mechanism which enables the body to make maximum use of a physiologically valuable group of substances. It may also be considered as a system for keeping in their place potentially harmful detergent materials. Its normal functioning depends on the harmonious working of numerous organs and on the controlling activity of both the nervous system and hormones. Its integrity is essential for health and its breakdown is attended by many ill-effects.

The enterohepatic circulation may be summed up as an endless flow of lipid-solvent from the liver by the biliary tract to the intestinal lumen and then back by the portal vein to the liver again. When the gallbladder is intact this flow is intermittent because it is initiated by the food-induced discharge of stored bile into the duodenum. It is halted or at least slowed by fasting.

Figure 6.1 shows the main events which occur during the entero-hepatic circulation. These are: addition to the circulating pool of newly synthesised primary bile salts, secretion into the biliary canaliculi, transport to the gallbladder for concentration and storage between meals, discharge into the duodenum resulting in mixture with chyme

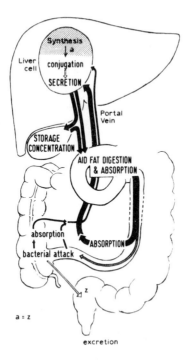

Fig. 6.1. The main events in the enterohepatic circulation.

and pancreatic juice, intimate involvement in lipid digestion and absorption, transport down the small intestine, absorption of the greater part by the special transport system in the ileum, partial deconjugation and dehydroxylation by intestinal bacteria, passive absorption by the colon (and perhaps terminal ileum) of some bacterially altered or secondary bile acids, transport in portal venous blood to the hepatocyte, uptake by the liver cell, reconjugation if necessary and finally re-secretion into the bile. All these events can probably take place two or three times during the digestion of a single meal.

The motive forces which keep this cycle moving are the liver cell's transport systems for taking up bile salts and secreting them into the bile, cholecystokinin-induced contraction of the gallbladder (with relaxation of the sphincter of Oddi), the propulsive movements of the small intestine, the active transport system in the ileal mucosa* and the flow of blood in the portal venous system. The normal operation of these forces results in bile salts being available in the right place at the right time and in the right concentration.

There are other substances which undergo some degree of entero-hepatic recirculation, such as urobilinogen, bilirubin, cholesterol and possibly fat-soluble vitamins and hormones. With all of these except cholesterol the recirculation is quantitatively and physiologically insignificant and, in the case of cholesterol, its movement is largely dependent on the operation of the bile salt cycle. Further, bile salt is probably the only recycled material which has its own special intestinal transport system. Such a mechanism is required to ensure the absorption of large polar molecules which are poorly transported by passive diffusion processes.

Each stage of the enterohepatic cycle will now be considered in greater detail.

HEPATIC UPTAKE AND SECRETION

Bile salts in the blood reaching the liver are taken up with great avidity. If isotopically labelled cholic acid is injected intravenously into normal subjects, half of it is removed from the systemic blood within 13 min [51, 351]. After it has been completely cleared, the radio-activity does not reappear in the systemic blood even though it is circulating enterohepatically in high concentration [51, 351]. In health the concentration of bile salts in fasting peripheral blood is so low (0.03-0.23 mg/100 ml, mean 0.08 [549]) that at least 99.7 per cent of the bile salt pool must be in the enterohepatic circuit. One hour after a meal the serum level is measurably but only slightly higher [549]. The equivalent concentration in human portal blood has not been estab-lished except in two patients with gastric cancer, in whom it was 12 and eight times higher than their peripheral blood levels [421]. In rats it has been reported as 60 μM [112] (or approximately 3.0 mg/100 ml) and as 200 μM [488] (or 10.0 mg/100 ml), in other words as 40-100 times higher than human peripheral blood levels. In cebus monkeys, portal

---

* The concentration gradient for deconjugated bile salts between intestinal lumen and blood is another factor promoting intestinal absorption but since it results in passive diffusion it is not to be considered a 'motive force'.

blood concentrations of bile salts varied up to 10 times higher than peripheral blood concentrations [526].

Direct measurements of the proportion of intravenously administered bile salt extracted in a single passage through the liver have given a figure of 92 per cent for taurocholate in dogs [493]. Glycocholate is probably extracted with equal efficiency even though the dog does not normally make glycine-conjugates, while free cholic acid is removed only slightly less efficiently [493].

These facts suggest that liver cells have a special transport mechanism for uptake of bile salts but little is known about it. Its capacity for transporting bile salt is certainly greater than that of the ileal transport system, at least in guinea-pigs [283] and rats [148]. Indeed in rats it has been estimated to be five times greater [148]. The total capacity of the liver to transport taurocholate into the bile has a saturation maximum [71, 277] but it is not known whether it is uptake or secretion which is the rate-limiting factor. Formal studies of uptake, storage and biliary Tm have not been reported and would be difficult to perform because large doses of bile salt given intravenously cause haemolysis. However, by analogy with BSP it is likely that the uptake mechanism has a greater capacity than the excretory one [696].

As with bilirubin, conjugation is virtually mandatory before bile salts are excreted into bile. Only in occasional individuals can free bile acids be detected in the bile, and then in very small amounts [267, 596]. Since free cholic acid is extracted from the blood almost as rapidly as its glycine and taurine conjugates (in the dog) [493] it is unlikely that conjugation is normally rate-limiting in bile salt transport. When there is exceptional demand for bile salt conjugation this may become a rate-limiting step, since patients who continually deconjugate most of their bile salts (ileal disorders and small bowel bacterial overgrowth) have high serum levels of free bile acids [394]. In these circumstances lack or unavailability of taurine and glycine side chains may be the limiting factor. In the dog, acute taurine depletion can be induced by infusing excessive amounts of cholic acid, and this does cause a fall in cholic acid transport across the liver. It also leads to the appearance of large amounts of unconjugated bile acid in the bile [491], but this is probably irrelevant to man since the dog is unable to conjugate with glycine [275].

It is generally accepted that secretion of bile salts into the canaliculi depends on a carrier-mediated active transport system [696]. The evidence is twofold. First, bile salt is excreted against an enormous concentration gradient between liver and bile. In the rat, the concentration of bile salts in liver tissue is only 0.14-0.28 mM [241], while in the bile it is 16 mM [363]. Second, the biliary excretory capacity can be saturated. The maximal excretory rate for taurocholate has been calculated in the dog as 8.5 μM/kg body weight/min and similar values were obtained for glycocholate [491], but no data are available for dihydroxy bile salts nor for excretory rates in man. The third of the classical criteria for active carrier-mediated transport, competition or mutual inhibition between pairs of transported compounds, has not been demonstrated for bile salts but has been for other actively transported anionic compounds. For example the oral cholecystographic agent iopanoic acid inhibits the biliary excretion of BSP [568]. It is likely that the bile salt transport system is different from that serving other organic anions since bile salts do not interfere with the maximal excretion of BSP [696] and may even enhance it [492]. Further, sheep with a hereditary defect of bilirubin excretion (bilirubin being another anion) have defective BSP transport but handle taurocholate normally [12]. Indeed a patient with the same defects of BSP and bilirubin transport (Dubin-Johnson syndrome) has been shown to have a normal bile salt excretion pattern [259].

In the act of crossing the canalicular membrane, or immediately thereafter, bile salts associate with phospholipid and cholesterol to form mixed micelles. The nature of this association is discussed in Chapter 3, and the relationship between bile salt secretion and the secretion of other biliary components is discussed in Chapter 8.

During their passage through the biliary tract bile salts are thought not to be absorbed to any significant extent, presumably because in their conjugated state they diffuse so slowly across biological membranes (see pages 69 and 74).

THE ROLE OF THE GALLBLADDER

During digestion it is presumed that the sphincter of Oddi remains relaxed and the gallbladder remains contracted so that freshly secreted bile is directed straight into the duodenum. However, during fasting most of the bile collects in the gallbladder and is concentrated there by removal of water and electrolytes, mainly through coupled active absorption of Na^+ and Cl^- [143]. Consequently the organic constituents of bile become concentrated by a factor of 5-10 times [129]. Assuming a gallbladder volume of 50 ml, this has the effect of making available for instant use at meal times a store of bile salts with the detergent power of 250-500 ml hepatic bile, which is the result of up to 12 hours secretory activity by the liver cells.

Little is known of the importance of this storage stage in the enterohepatic cycle. One way of evaluating it is to study the effects of cholecystectomy. Judged by the crude criterion of faecal fat excretion, cholecystectomy does not interfere significantly with fat absorption [372] (except in dogs after ileectomy, a procedure which may magnify the importance of the gallbladder's reservoir function [342]). Presumably therefore it does not cause serious bile salt depletion. After cholecystectomy, the concentration of bile salt in the intestine during digestion is not obviously low and the incorporation of lipid into the micellar phase is normal [66]. Isotope dilution studies [517] indicate that in patients without a gallbladder the bile salt pool is only occasionally smaller than in matched controls, and that this pool is metabolised but not turned over more rapidly than normal (see Chapter 14). (In hypercholesterolaemic patients [707] and in dogs [706] there is some evidence for a small pool size and rapid turnover of bile salts after cholecystectomy.) A priori there is no reason to expect the pool to be reduced after cholecystectomy since rats, which lack a gallbladder, maintain a pool which is at least as large relative to body weight as that of rodents which do have a gallbladder (see page 174).

Besides receiving, storing and concentrating bile, the function of the gallbladder is to react to the stimulus of eating by contracting and discharging its contents into the duodenum. Within 30 min of eating [594], or within 10 min of intravenous cholecystokinin injection [669], there is normally a sharp rise in duodenal bile salt concentration. No such peak occurs after cholecystectomy [669]. In contracting, the gallbladder acts as a motor driving the enterohepatic circulation [410]. When the gallbladder is inert, as it is in many patients with coeliac disease, the half-life of radioactive taurocholate is much longer than normal, probably because bile salts are sequestered in a sterile part of the enterohepatic circuit. There is in effect a sluggish enterohepatic circulation [410].

Absorption of bile salts by the gallbladder does not normally take place to any significant extent, presumably because conjugated bile salts are poorly transported by the only mechanism available, passive diffusion. However, guinea-pig experiments [495] suggest that significant absorption of bile salts can occur in two situations: (a) if the gallbladder mucosa is damaged, and (b) if deconjugation takes place as a result of bacterial infection, in which case the free bile acids, especially the least polar or dihydroxy ones, diffuse out quite readily. These facts provide ammunition for the dwindling army of believers in an infective origin of gallstones.

THE INTESTINAL PHASE

This is the crucial stage in the life history of bile salts. It is in the intestine that bile salts play their major physiological role and that their own fate is decided. For purposes of discussion it is useful to distinguish an upper and a lower intestinal phase.

The *upper intestinal phase* is a period of intensive physicochemical activity concerned with the digestion and absorption of lipids. The details of this explosive process are considered in Chapters 8 and 3. It takes place mainly in the duodenum and upper jejunum. By the end of the jejunum most if not all of the lipids and other nutrients have been absorbed but most if not all of the bile salts remain within the lumen [56, 59, 60]. This is because conjugated bile salt molecules are too large and polar to be absorbed except by a special transport system which is found only in the ileum. Bile salts probably emerge from the jejunum quite unaltered chemically. The scarcity of bacteria in the upper intestine makes it unlikely that any significant breakdown occurs, and for practical purposes free bile acids are not found in the jejunum of normal subjects. Physicochemically, bile salts remain in micellar solution since their concentration remains over 2 mM throughout the small intestine [191, 594]. As the products of lipolysis are absorbed the micelles presumably shrink and come to contain bile salts and little if anything else.

The *lower intestinal phase* is the most fateful part of the enterohepatic circulation as far as the bile salts themselves are concerned. It takes place in the ileum and proximal colon. Here one of three possible fates awaits each bile salt molecule—to be absorbed unchanged, to be absorbed but in a changed form, or to be excreted. In this complex and ever-changing situation there are five main factors to be considered:

 (1) The intestinal flora.

 (2) The physicochemical properties of the various bile acids.

(3) The unabsorbed dietary residue.
(4) The rate of intestinal transit.
(5) The properties of the absorptive mechanisms.

These factors interact in various ways, but it is helpful to consider separately how each affects the physical and chemical states of bile salts and their availability for absorption.

THE INTESTINAL FLORA AND ITS EFFECTS ON BILE SALTS

The recent burst of interest in human intestinal flora springs to some extent from the realisation that bacteria have profound effects upon bile salts and that these effects are sometimes of clinical significance. The conditions necessary for bacterial attack to occur seem to be a total count of over $10^4/mm^3$ and the presence of obligate anaerobes [159, 227]. In the normal small intestine, anaerobes in large numbers are not found except in the most terminal part of the ileum, just proximal to the ileo-caecal sphincter [226]. This is also the only part of the small gut where bacterially altered bile acids are found.

The changes produced by intestinal bacteria fall into two classes:

(a) Changes which may be followed by absorption of the altered bile acids. These are deconjugation and 7α-dehydroxylation.
(b) Changes which are not followed by absorption. These are oxidation, reduction and epimerisation.

Changes in class (b) obviously affect the pattern of bile salts in the faeces but not that in the bile. Therefore we are only concerned at this point with class (a) changes.

Deconjugation is the most thoroughly studied of the bacterial alterations. A number of different organisms are capable of this hydrolytic process *in vitro*, including enterococci, clostridia, bacteroides, bifidobacteria, Streptococcus faecalis and veillonella (for references see Aries & Hill [13] and Shimada *et al.* [582]). What is important is that most species of bacteroides and bifidobacterium have this capacity, since these anaerobes comprise the vast majority of human colonic bacteria [224]. There is probably no significant difference in the rate at which different bile salts are split [158, 582], though exceptions have been reported [432, 582]. The enzyme responsible for deconjugation is called cholanylglycine hydrolase [13]. Being partly extracellular, it is found in solution in intestinal contents

[485] and can be extracted from Clostridia in pure form for laboratory use [467]. It is probable that *in vivo* this enzyme is optimally active under anaerobic conditions [13].

The extent to which deconjugation occurs in normal subjects was not appreciated until studies were made of the fate of radioactively labelled bile salts. Such studies suggested that each day up to one third of the bile salt pool is deconjugated [214, 480], but the most recent work indicates that no less than 8-21 per cent of the glycocholate pool is deconjugated at each enterohepatic cycle [294a].

The site at which deconjugation occurs has not been definitely established. It is often assumed that it is limited to the colon, perhaps because in an early study Sjövall found no free bile acids in the ileal aspirates of two subjects [594]. However, in one recent study free bile acids were found 'consistently' in the terminal ileum [486] and in another they were present in four of 11 normal subjects [98]. Also patients with ileostomies show a normal or even increased rate of deconjugation of labelled taurocholate [454]. It is probable therefore that under normal conditions a significant amount of deconjugation does occur in the terminal ileum.

The glycine released by deconjugation is largely absorbed and metabolised. Radioactive studies show that about half of it ends up as CO_2 in expired air [294a].

7α-Dehydroxylation results in the conversion of cholate to deoxycholate and of chenodeoxycholate to lithocholate (see Fig. 2.7, page 19). It has not been studied extensively until the last few years. In 1968 Hill & Drasar [297] showed that a few strains of bacteroides, clostridium, veillonella and streptococcus faecalis from the human intestine possessed the ability to convert cholate to deoxycholate, and in the same year Midtvedt & Norman [443] reported that an anaerobic lactobacillus (bifidobacterium) from rat faeces would dehydroxylate both cholate and chenodeoxycholate. Thus it is likely that the same bacteria are responsible for forming both deoxycholate and lithocholate. In the rat at least, these bacteria are restricted to the large intestine [434]. In man, too, dehydroxylation seems to be a special function of the colon, since ileostomy patients have little or no deoxycholate in their bile or intestinal effluent [438, 454, 508]. This may, however, reflect only a shorter or less intense contact between the bile salts and the appropriate bacteria, since ileostomy effluent does contain a considerable number of bacteroides [225]. Another condition for 7α-dehydroxylation to take place is that deconjugation should take place first [433, 480] which, in the rat at least, means that there must be separate deconjugating bacteria present [253]. The bacteria which remove the 7α-hydroxyl group are capable of oxidising it too [252, 253].

The extent to which dehydroxylation occurs in normal man is not precisely known. In rats half the cholic acid pool is dehydroxylated each day [405]. The figure for man is certainly much less. In four gallstone patients, Norman [480] found 3-6 per cent of the glyco-cholate pool was recirculated in dehydroxylated form after 24 h. After a normal subject's bile salt pool is labelled with taurocholate—24-^{14}C, each day the proportion of total biliary radioactivity in the deoxy-cholates increases by about 10 per cent [214, 278].

The reaction of 7α-dehydroxylation is of interest clinically because of the well-known toxicity of deoxycholate, and especially of litho-cholate (see Chapter 9).

Other Bacterial Effects on Bile Acids (Class (b) Changes)

The other transformations undergone during passage through the colon include oxidation of the C-3, C-7 and C-12 hydroxyl groups to form keto bile acids, and reduction of these keto groups to yield both α-hydroxy and β-hydroxy epimers. Some of the organisms and enzymes responsible for these reactions have been identified and studied [14, 432]. As a result of their activities, and of others including 6β-hydroxy-lation and the formation of 5α- or allo- derivatives, the faecal bile acid mixture is extremely complex [37]. At a recent count it consisted of not less than 30 compounds [122]. Some of these are acylated with fatty acid at the 3 position [481], which must make them very insoluble [307].

From studies in five subjects, it seems that the main faecal end products of cholic acid are deoxycholate and 12-keto-lithocholate, while those of chenodeoxycholic acid are lithocholate and iso-litho-cholate [124, 479].

In spite of this extensive metabolism it is still generally accepted that the steroid ring of bile acids remains intact during passage through the intestine [307] (a fact which has even aroused anxiety regarding the possibility of steroid pollution of the environment through disposal of human faeces! [314]. The role of bacteria in binding bile acids is discussed on page 71.

THE EFFECT OF BACTERIAL TRANSFORMATIONS ON THE ENTEROHEPATIC CIRCULATION

The overall significance of bacteria can presumably be deduced by comparing the normal with the germ-free animal. Germ-free and chemotherapeutically treated rats recirculate their bile acids more efficiently than normal, their cholic acid half-life being 10-15 days, compared with two days in control animals [251, 256, 404, 521]. These changes were first noted in rats on synthetic, low-residue diets and the difference is much less marked on ordinary rat food [256]. Nevertheless it seems certain that, in rats at least, the normal intestinal flora promotes the excretion of bile salts. The mechanism of this effect is not entirely clear. Certainly bile acids tend to adsorb to bacteria [254, 255], but more importantly binding to any solid matter is greater after deconjugation and dehydroxylation [167, 255].

Deconjugation alone is not enough to explain why normal rats excrete bile salts so much more rapidly than germ-free ones, since mono-contamination of a germ-free animal with a deconjugating micro-organism makes no difference to the total faecal excretion of bile salts or their half-life, even though the faeces contain free bile acids [251, 353]. It cannot even be said that dehydroxylation is the critical step determining whether the result of a bile salt-bacterium interaction is excretion or reabsorption, since the rabbit, which keeps all its bile salts in the dehydroxylated form (as deoxycholate), recirculates them for a longer time than does man, in whom only about 20 per cent of the pool is dehydroxylated [292]. In man himself, the increased rate of dehydroxylation present after cholecystectomy is not associated with more rapid excretion of bile salts [517].

It is possible that the effect of bacteria on bile acid excretion is part of a more general effect on intestinal function. Gustafsson & Norman [256] have suggested that bacteria influence the intestinal transit rate. They found that germ-free rats pass carmine markers very slowly on a synthetic diet but at a normal rate on a fibre-containing pelleted diet, and at the same time the half-life of cholic acid was greatly prolonged on the synthetic diet but only slightly prolonged on the pelleted diet. This by itself suggests that the transit rate is more important than the bacterial flora in determining the fate of bile acids. However, in conventional rats the synthetic diet caused only slight slowing of the transit rate and of cholic acid turnover. In effect the presence of intestinal bacteria counteracted the transit-slowing effect of a synthetic diet, which is tantamount to saying that the intestinal bacteria in some way promote intestinal transit.

There are unfortunately no studies in man which allow generalisations about the overall role of bacteria in the human enterohepatic cycle.

THE PHYSICOCHEMICAL PROPERTIES OF BILE ACIDS IN RELATION TO THEIR CHANCES OF ABSORPTION OR EXCRETION

Two properties must be considered—solubility and polarity.

For any substance to be absorbed it has to be present in the intestinal lumen in aqueous solution (ignoring the now discredited idea of pinocytosis). At the pH of the terminal ileum, probably about 8, all the six main conjugated bile salts are freely soluble, and free cholate, deoxycholate and chenodeoxycholate are quite soluble. All these bile salts should therefore be well absorbed if they make contact with an absorptive surface. Lithocholate and its conjugates are, however, very insoluble and so much less likely to be absorbed.

The less polar a bile salt is, the more likely is it to bind to unabsorbed plant fibre or to bacteria, but also the more easily is it absorbed by passive diffusion. Polarity is determined by two factors: (a) the number of hydroxyl groups on the nucleus and (b) the degree of ionisation of the acid or carboxyl group. The degree of ionisation, as predicted by the pK_a of the acid, is greatest for the taurine conjugates, intermediate for the glycine conjugates and least for the free acids. Thus the main bile salts can be placed in descending order of polarity as follows: taurocholate, taurochenodeoxy- and taurodeoxycholate*, (taurolithocholate), glycocholate, glycochenodeoxy- and glycodeoxycholate*, cholate, (glycolithocholate), chenodeoxycholate, deoxycholate, lithocholate. This polar hierarchy is perhaps best understood by examining a thin-layer chromatogram (Fig. 6.2) in which it can be seen that the less polar a bile salt, the faster it runs.

* The conjugated chenodeoxycholates are marginally more polar than the conjugated deoxycholates.

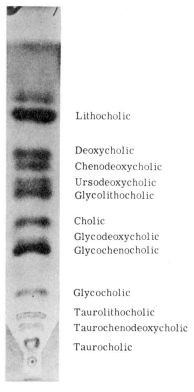

Lithocholic

Deoxycholic
Chenodeoxycholic
Ursodeoxycholic
Glycolithocholic

Cholic
Glycodeoxycholic
Glycochenocholic

Glycocholic

Taurolithocholic

Taurochenodeoxycholic

Taurocholic

Fig. 6.2. An ascending thin-layer chromatogram of a mixture of 12 bile acids showing separation in order of polarity (least polar at the top). Taurodeoxycholic acid is not shown as it is inseparable from taurochenodeoxycholic acid. Ursodeoxycholic acid is a stereoisomer of chenodeoxycholic acid, present in many mammals. From Gregg [239].

THE UNABSORBED DIETARY RESIDUE

This is a factor which is completely neglected in most discussions of intestinal absorption, giving one the impression that the average person lives on a synthetic formula diet! Nevertheless the dietary residue may be of great importance. It is made up almost entirely of the structural polysaccharides of plants. The main components of this vegetable fibre are cellulose, hemi-celluloses or pentosans, and lignin. They are important in determining the fate of bile acids for two reasons: (a) they modify intestinal motility and absorption in general; (b) they provide binding sites for bile acids.

Adding fibre to the diet has been shown to increase the excretion of bile acids. In rats, adding 20 per cent cellulose to a synthetic diet brought down the half-life of cholic acid from 4.17 days to 1.44 days and trebled the faecal excretion of labelled bile acids [525]. In young Indian girls adding large amounts of cellulose to the diet increased faecal bile acids significantly [584]. Subjects on a high fibre diet excreted more bile acids than those on a low fibre diet [10].

Eastwood & Boyd [164] have thrown some light on these phenomena by showing that cellulose enrichment of the rat's diet increases the concentration of bile acids in both the fluid and the sediment of the small intestine including the ileum. This suggests that fibre keeps bile acids within the intestinal lumen, both by trapping dissolved ones in the interstices of the fibrous bulk and by reducing the amount in solution. The latter effect has been attributed to binding of bile acids, and *in vitro* the lignin component of vegetable fibre has been shown to have quite potent bile acid binding properties [167]. This binding is most effective with the least polar bile acids, which suggests hydrophobic rather than ionic binding. In man, lignin-enrichment of the diet does not accelerate the excretion of radioactive taurocholate or its circulating metabolites [282]. This makes it unlikely that lignin by itself is responsible for the effect of fibre on bile acid excretion, which may be due entirely to the physical trapping of bile salts, together with the well-known effect of dietary roughage in accelerating intestinal transit. If any binding of bile salts does occur it will certainly involve lithocholate because of its low polarity.

This effect of dietary fibre may be of great clinical significance. There are reasons to link the consumption of fibre-depleted foods with metabolic disorders (hypercholesterolaemia and gallstones) in which there may be under-excretion of bile acids (see pages 156, 171 and 188).

BINDING BY BACTERIA

Bile acids are bound by bacteria. This has been well shown in rats, in which 27-44 per cent of the caecal bile acids are normally attached to solid matter, but none at all if the rats are germ-free [254, 255]. *In vitro* experiments [482] and stool analyses [479] suggest that, to be tightly bound in this way, bile acids must be less polar than deoxycholic acid, which remains for the most part in solution or at least dialysable [255, 482]. Lithocholic acid is strongly bound by bacteria [252, 482]. It is unlikely that significant bacterial binding occurs in the small intestine of man, since it is absent from that of the coprophagic rat [254], but in the colon it is probably a major factor preventing reabsorption of degraded bile acids.

THE RATE OF INTESTINAL TRANSIT

To be absorbed, bile acids must make contact with an absorptive epithelium and presumably the chances of such contact occurring depend to some extent on the transit rate. Nevertheless this relationship has scarcely been investigated. The studies on dietary fibre and bulk mentioned above, especially those on germ-free rats [256], strongly suggest that transit rate is a limiting factor in bile salt absorption, but the motility effects of dietary residue are hard to separate from its trapping and binding effects. The ideal experiment, in which transit rate is controllably increased without altering the luminal milieu, is yet to be performed. Meihoff & Kern [426] approached the problem by feeding volunteers mannitol in doses large enough to cause diarrhoea, and they did show a substantial increase in bile acid excretion. However, this experiment must have involved a marked dilution of the intestinal contents. In patients with malabsorption due to the carcinoid syndrome, pharmacological control of the diarrhoea sometimes reduces steatorrhoea [430], while in dogs with bypass of most of the small intestine insertion of an anti-peristaltic segment decreases not only transit rate but also faecal fat and nitrogen [620]. These facts suggest that abnormally rapid transit interferes with absorption in general, and so probably with bile salt absorption.

The effects of abnormally slow transit are also largely unexplored. The prolonged recirculation of radiocholate in rats on a synthetic fibre-free diet [525] suggests that slow transit allows super-normal absorption of bile salts. However, excessive slowing to the extent of stagnation allows proliferation of faecal-type bacteria in the small intestine, and this probably disrupts the enterohepatic circulation (see Chapter 10).

THE PROPERTIES OF THE ABSORPTIVE MECHANISMS

The mechanisms available for absorbing bile acids are:

(a) A specialised transport system. This is present only in the ileum, and is maximally active in the distal quarter of the small intestine [376].

(b) Non-specific passive absorption. This is possible through any part of the small or large intestine, since it depends only on movement down a concentration or, more precisely, electro-chemical gradient. The only limiting factor is the permeability of the absorptive membrane.

These two mechanisms will now be considered in turn.

THE ILEAL TRANSPORT SYSTEM

The discovery of this system in 1961 by Lack & Weiner [375] caused great interest because, apart from vitamin B_{12}, no other nutritionally important substance has a special absorptive mechanism in the ileum, and also because it makes attractively good sense to delay bile salt absorption until after dietary lipids have been absorbed.

A good deal of *in vitro* work has established that this has all the credentials demanded of an active transport system [148, 319, 375, 512]. It can transport bile salts uphill, that is against an electrochemical gradient, though in life this is never necessary. It demonstrates its dependence on cellular energy by ceasing to function when deprived of oxygen, or poisoned with inhibitors of metabolism. It shows that it has a limited number of carrier sites by having a maximum velocity of transport, or V_{max} (so-called saturation kinetics). The existence of mutual inhibition between pairs of bile salts [283, 320, 378] confirms this latter point since it implies competition for transport sites. This phenomenon also supports the idea that there is a common transport system for all naturally occurring bile salts [378]. Pursuing this line of reasoning to a more theoretical level, it has been shown by using a variety of artificial bile salts, that to be available for transport a bile salt must have a negative charge on the side chain [378], and possibly a hydroxyl group on the nucleus [561].

Different bile salts are transported by this system at different rates. Tri-hydroxy bile salts, free or conjugated, are transported 6-8 times faster than di-hydroxy and about 10 times faster than mono-hydroxy. Furthermore, the affinity of bile salts for the transport carriers is 4-6 times greater for conjugated salts than for free ones [561]. This implies that free bile salts cannot compete effectively for active transport [561]. Taurine conjugates are probably absorbed more efficiently than glycine conjugates [196]. In summary, the active transport system is ideally adapted for extracting taurocholate and glycocholate from the intestinal lumen, and it can also efficiently absorb the taurine and glycine di-hydroxy conjugates. (The chances of transport of the di-hydroxy conjugates are increased by the fact that they compete effectively with the tri-hydroxy conjugates for absorption [283, 320, 378].)

PASSIVE ABSORPTION

It is a general property of biological membranes that they are much less permeable to ionised acids and bases than to unionised materials. Ions are able to diffuse across if the electrical gradient is favourable, which it is for acids (anions) in the intestine since the inner side of the bowel wall is negatively charged. However, passive ionic diffusion is a much slower process than passive non-ionic diffusion. For a bile salt (cholate), non-ionic diffusion was over seven times faster than ionic diffusion *in vitro* and nearly six times faster *in vivo*, using rat jejunum [148]. The extent to which these two processes occur will vary with the luminal pH and with the different bile salts since they have different pK_a values. At pH 8 virtually all the free and conjugated bile salts are in the ionised form and so in the ileum it is unlikely that significant non-ionic diffusion takes place.* At pH 6, as found in the jejunum, half of the free bile acids and a fraction of the glycine conjugates are unionised and available for non-ionic diffusion. However, free bile acids are not normally found in the jejunum.

Another factor affecting polarity and therefore the rate of diffusion is the number of hydroxyl groups on the steroid nucleus. For example taurodeoxycholate (two hydroxyl groups) is absorbed from the rat's jejunum three times as fast as taurocholate, and taurolithocholate (one hydroxyl group) 10 times as fast [609], while in the guinea-pig free chenodeoxycholate is absorbed from the jejunum much faster than free cholate [412]. In general therefore bile salts which are absorbed less well by the active transport system are absorbed better by passive diffusion and vice versa.

There is considerable species variation in the permeability of the intestinal mucosa to bile salts. The rat and the dog have far more

* In support of this statement, simultaneous analyses of the bile acid pattern in intestinal contents and portal blood have shown no preferential absorption of free bile acids [112].

permeable jejunums than the rabbit, spider monkey and guinea-pig, as judged by the *in vivo* absorption of taurocholate [221, 690]. The situation in man is unknown.

Dietschy has suggested a further mechanism for bile salt absorption, namely diffusion of intact micelles across the mucosa [145] (or possibly disintegration at the mucosal surface [562]). The evidence for this is that micellar solutions of taurodeoxycholate (20 molecules per micelle) are absorbed faster then micellar solutions of taurocholate (four molecules per micelle) [609] and also that the diffusion rate increases disproportionately when the concentration is raised above the CMC [562]. However, Gibaldi has suggested a different interpretation of these facts, namely that the higher diffusion rates reflect only increased permeability of the mucosa brought about by the bile salts themselves [219]. If the taurocholate micelles are expanded by adding a second amphiphile, such as phospholipid, so producing bulky mixed micelles (or alternatively reducing the permeability effect on the mucosa), then the rate of diffusion is much retarded [609]. This mechanism could provide an additional explanation for the minimal absorption of conjugated bile salts in the jejunum *in vivo*.

Possible contributions to the absorption of bile salts by solvent drag, exchange diffusion and facilitated diffusion have been discussed and ruled out [145].

RELATIVE CONTRIBUTIONS OF THE JEJUNUM AND ILEUM, AND OF ACTIVE AND PASSIVE TRANSPORT TO TOTAL BILE SALT ABSORPTION

It is generally agreed that, thanks to the active transport system, the ileum is a much more efficient organ for bile salt absorption than the jejunum. This superiority has been repeatedly demonstrated by experiments in which bile salts have been placed in tied-off jejunal and ileal loops of various animals and have disappeared from the lumen faster or appeared in the bile faster when ileal loops were used [21, 148, 202, 221, 631, 648, 663, 687, 690]. This suggests that the main physiological site of bile salt absorption is the ileum. However, in some of these experiments conjugated bile salts did disappear from jejunal loops at a significant rate [21, 148, 202, 648, 687], and in experiments when free cholate was used it did appear in the bile at a significant rate [148, 631, 663]. These facts, together with the very rapid appearance of orally administered bile salts in the bile of bile-fistula animals [238, 599], have been interpreted by some as meaning that substantial proximal passive absorption of bile salts takes place, and that the role of the ileum is merely to deal efficiently with 'stragglers'.

The evidence for this idea does not stand up to critical examination.

(1) The results of keeping pure bile salt solutions in contact with short, washed-out intestinal segments for 1 or 2 h may not be the same as what happens in physiological circumstances in the upper small bowel. It is known, for example, that bile salts are less well absorbed from micelles expanded with lipid than from pure bile salt micelles [145].

(2) In rats during digestion the intraluminal bile salt concentration stays constant or even rises throughout the jejunum [145, 164]. The same is probably true of man [594].

(3) Disappearance from the lumen is not conclusive evidence of absorption, and may represent only adsorption to the brush border of the epithelial cells. There is evidence that uptake of bile salts can be followed by release and return to the jejunal lumen [440].

(4) Appearance in the bile is of course proof of absorption. However, its demonstration with free cholate is physiologically irrelevant since free bile salts are not normally present in the jejunum in significant amounts. Evidence that true absorption of conjugated bile salts occurs from the jejunum to a significant extent is lacking.

(5) In rats [145] and men [588], perfusion experiments using an unabsorbable marker have shown that taurocholate disappears very slowly from the jejunal lumen.

(6) In dogs whose bile had been labelled with radioactive taurocholate, resection of the ileum caused the label to disappear almost completely after one meal, whereas resection of the jejunum had no effect [513]. This shows firstly that the jejunum is unnecessary for taurocholate absorption, secondly that the ileum is very necessary, and thirdly that the jejunum can do very little in the absence of the ileum to maintain an enterohepatic circulation.

(7) Similarly, in man studies with radioactive bile salts have shown that resection or disease of the ileum causes such rapid disappearance of labelled bile salts [426, 622] as to constitute a virtual breakdown of the enterohepatic circulation [17, 280].

In the light of this evidence it seems improbable that the jejunum plays a significant part in normal bile salt absorption. There is, however, persuasive evidence from jejunal perfusion studies in man [298, 639] that glycine conjugates, especially of the di-hydroxy bile acids, can (thanks to their relatively low polarity) be absorbed to some extent proximally by non-ionic diffusion.* These studies are subject to the limitations mentioned in points (1) and (3), but have been widely accepted as applicable to the physiological situation. Proponents of this view may dismiss points (5) and (6) as not necessarily relevant to glycine conjugates, and may point out that the bile radioactivity studies of point (7) magnify any defect in absorption since, to be valid, specific activity measurements in duodenal aspirates must be made at intervals of not less than 24 h [313], which allows at least six recirculations to take place. They may also quote experiments with rhesus monkeys giving indirect evidence that resection of the distal small intestine leaves intact 50 per cent of the bile absorption mechanism [154]. Against these findings must be placed the results of direct attacks on the problem in man. These showed that, in ileectomy patients, 95 per cent or more of labelled glycine conjugates are lost from the enterohepatic circulation after a single meal [411]. In a separate study, labelled cholic acid was excreted in the faeces as fast as a non-absorbable marker [709]. If glycine conjugates are absorbed proximally, there should be a fall in the ratio of glycine to taurine conjugates in distal intestinal aspirates even in normal subjects. The limited data available show no evidence of such a fall [594, 645]. It seems very desirable that further studies of this type should be made in which a non-absorbable marker is used and all the individual bile salt fractions are measured, but in the meantime it must be stated that the balance of evidence is against significant jejunal absorption of bile salts.†

Doubt has been thrown on the pre-eminence of the ileal active

---

* Perfusion through a 50 cm segment resulted in disappearance of 24.5 per cent of the glycine conjugates (di-hydroxy more than tri-hydroxy), compared with 3.3 per cent of taurine conjugates and 60.0 per cent of free bile acids [298].

† The related controversy over the mechanism of the high G/T ratio in patients with ileal disorders is discussed in Chapter 10.

transport system by the suggestion that in the terminal ileum there is considerable absorption of deconjugated bile salts by passive non-ionic diffusion [145, 486]. This may be so provided (a) there is extensive bacterial deconjugation of bile salts in the terminal ileum, and (b) the pH in the lumen is such that free bile acids are present in a non-ionised state. There is at present inadequate information on the extent of deconjugation in the terminal ileum. However, studies of the fate of circulating radioactive taurocholate have indicated that the taurine moiety is lost slowly over several days in most normal subjects [214, 278]. This implies that for the most part taurocholate, and therefore presumably the other bile salts, are absorbed intact. The pH in the terminal ileum is generally between 7.3 and 7.8 [191]. At this pH even the free bile acids are largely ionised. If the unionised fraction were absorbed quickly, this would perhaps keep the equilibrium reaction $HA \rightleftharpoons H^+ + A^-$ moving to the left and so constitute an effective absorptive mechanism. It may even be that free bile acids in the terminal ileum depend on passive absorption because their access to active transport carriers is blocked by the more avidly taken up conjugated bile salts [145]. However, it must be emphasised that deconjugation is not necessary for efficient bile salt absorption, since germ-free and antibiotic-treated rats recirculate their bile salts more, not less, efficiently than normal [251, 404]. Furthermore, studies of portal bile acid patterns give no support to the idea that free bile acids are absorbed more efficiently than conjugated ones [112].

In summary, taurine conjugates are absorbed exclusively in the terminal ileum by the active transport system; glycine conjugates, though theoretically absorbable by passive non-ionic diffusion at all levels, are also highly dependent on the ileal transport system; and any free bile acids in the small intestine are probably absorbed mainly by passive non-ionic diffusion, most rapidly in areas with lower pH.

THE ROLE OF THE COLON IN BILE SALT ABSORPTION

If carried past the ileo-caecal valve, bile salts can be absorbed from the colon but to a limited extent. Because of the enormous bacterial population in the colon, only free bile acids are present there in significant amounts. The main mechanism for their absorption is non-ionic passive diffusion. Injection of labelled free bile acids into the rat's colon is followed by slow but significant absorption [631], and when ^{14}C-labelled cholic, deoxycholic and 7-keto-deoxycholic acids were injected into the rat caecum about half were recovered from a bile fistula [483]. Rather surprisingly, germ-free rats absorb labelled glycocholate and taurocholate to the same extent as cholic acid [257]. This suggests that, given time, passive ionic diffusion can make a significant contribution. In germ-free rats, lithocholate was absorbed well too, presumably because there were no bacteria to bind it [257]. In dogs, perfusion of the entire colon with a solution containing free bile acids resulted in 7.3 per cent absorption of cholic acid, 16.7 per cent absorption of deoxycholic acid and 18.7 per cent absorption of chenodeoxycholic acid [427].

Recently it has been shown that the human colon has a significant capacity for absorbing bile acids. In eight patients undergoing biliary tract surgery, cholic acid-24-^{14}C was injected into the colon at laparotomy [548]. Bile collected by T-tube drainage over the next five days contained on average 59 per cent of the administered radio-activity, mostly in dehydroxylated form as deoxycholate. Using the same technique, we have obtained almost identical results in four patients and have also shown substantial absorption of labelled taurocholate in two patients, again appearing in the bile mainly in the form of deoxycholate [453]. In total colon perfusion studies, Mekhjian et al. have demonstrated substantial absorption of free and conjugated bile acids [428].

While the above studies prove that the colon can absorb bile acids under certain artificial conditions, they do no more than suggest that it does so in the normal state. The strongest evidence that it does is the presence in normal bile of deoxycholate, since this secondary bile salt is virtually absent from the bile of patients with total procto-colectomy [438, 454, 508].

The quantitative significance of colonic absorption is impossible to assess. After discussing the various estimates in the literature, Weiner & Lack [691] concluded: '. . . it is obvious that absorption from the large bowel, while important, represents only a small fraction (3-15 per cent) of the total enterohepatic circulation in the normal rat'. The same statement could probably be made of normal man. Indeed since man, unlike the rat, has a gallbladder in which his bile salts are protected from incessant exposure to intestinal bacteria, it is perhaps likely that his colon is called upon to play less part in bile salt absorption than is that of the rat.

THE ROLE OF THE ILEO-CAECAL SPHINCTER

The ileo-caecal sphincter is a poorly understood structure but if, like other sphincters, it serves to control the forward passage of alimentary contents and to prevent their reflux backwards, its function must be important to the integrity of the enterohepatic circulation. In dog experiments, removal of the sphincter has exaggerated the weight loss and steatorrhoea which follow ileal resection [242, 371, 590], increased the bacterial population of the small intestine [242], and had variable effects on intestinal transit time [242, 590]. Resection of the ileo-caecal sphincter alone has not been adequately studied but there is some evidence that it leads to bacterial overpopulation of the terminal ileum [216].

If ileo-caecal incompetence occurs in man, and radiologists would unhesitatingly say that it does, it may well upset the enterohepatic circulation, either by allowing too rapid transit through the terminal ileum and so bile salt malabsorption, or by allowing excessive bacterial breakdown of bile salts in the ileum. These events certainly occur in structural disease of the ileo-caecal region, for example Crohn's disease [214, 426], and probably occur in patients with surgical anastomosis of the small bowel to the colon. The latter point is, however, poorly documented.

It is possible that similar events occur as a functional abnormality in 'normal' subjects. In studies in this department of taurocholate-24-^{14}C turnover and metabolism we have unexpectedly come across two normal subjects who have lost half their labelled bile salt in under one day, and two normal subjects who deconjugated most or all of their taurocholate within 24 h (unpublished data). It is tempting to suggest that some cases of 'functional diarrhoea' may be due to ileo-caecal incompetence and its effects on bile salt metabolism, especially since it has been reported that oral administration of cholestyramine relieves the diarrhoea of some patients with the irritable bowel syndrome [558].

RETURN OF ABSORBED BILE SALTS TO THE LIVER

After absorption, bile salts are carried in the portal blood to the liver [599], probably bound to serum albumin [543]. Portal blood is difficult to obtain and rather few studies have been made of its bile acid pattern [112, 489]. In the rat 10-35 per cent of the portal bile acids are deconjugated, depending on the diet (the lower figure being obtained on a semi-synthetic diet) [112]. The pattern of bile acids in portal blood exactly resembled that found in the intestine [112]. No human data on portal bile acids are available but would clearly be of great interest, especially in relation to lithocholate. Recent studies have shown cholic acid to be bound by plasma albumin more strongly than taurocholate [78]. This may mean that binding is inversely related to polarity, in which case deoxycholate would be bound more strongly than cholate, and lithocholate more strongly still. How this would affect hepatic uptake is unknown.

On arrival back at the liver, bile salts are taken up as described earlier. Deconjugated bile acids are reconjugated. Dehydroxylated bile acids remain as such in man, but are largely re-hydroxylated in rats and mice [37, 405].

SUMMARY OF THE ENTEROHEPATIC CIRCULATION

Conjugated bile salts are secreted into the bile by a special transport mechanism and stored in the gallbladder. When food is taken, bile salts enter the duodenum in high concentration, pass down the small intestine and are reabsorbed mainly in the terminal ileum. Anaerobic bacteria in the ileum and colon deconjugate a significant proportion of the bile salt pool, and bacteria in the colon dehydroxylate a lesser proportion before reabsorption occurs. The chances of a bile salt being absorbed are affected by its polarity and solubility, by the presence of food residue and by the intestinal transit rate. All bile salts can be absorbed by active transport in the ileum, but the most efficiently transported bile salts are the most polar ones. The converse is true of passive absorption. Absorbed bile salts return in the portal vein and, if necessary, are re-conjugated before being re-secreted into the bile. Unabsorbed bile salts are further degraded in the colon before being excreted in the faeces.

7 Bile Salts in Motion: The Kinetics of the Enterohepatic Circulation and Homeostatic Mechanisms

After the qualitative description of the enterohepatic cycle in Chapter 6 the present chapter concerns its quantitative aspects. This is most easily done on the basis of a model of the enterohepatic circulation, shown in Fig. 7.1. The wheel represents a circulating pool which is continually

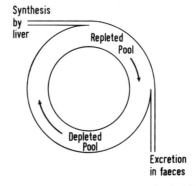

Fig. 7.1. A simple model of the enterohepatic circulation (after Hofmann [306]).

depleted by faecal excretion and repleted by hepatic synthesis. Over a period of time synthesis must be equal to excretion; otherwise the pool would steadily increase or decrease in size. It is a reasonable (but untested) assumption that the size of the pool, indicated in the model by the width of the wheel, does not vary materially from day to day, and therefore that daily synthesis equals daily excretion. It is quite possible that excretion is not immediately compensated by synthesis, so that some of the bile salts lost in the formation of faeces by day are not replaced until the overnight fast. However, limited data suggest that the bile salt pool is no smaller in the evening than in the morning [673].

Currently accepted ideas about the normal bile salt pool are that it is 2-4 g in size, that it circulates twice with each meal, and that each day it loses and is repleted with 500-700 mg or about 15-20 per cent of the total. Evidence for these statements is presented and discussed later in this chapter. Assuming they are true, it may be calculated that for a three-meal day, up to 24 g of bile salts enter and perfuse the small intestine each day, that the efficiency of intestinal absorption is about 97 per cent and that each bile salt molecule enters the intestine on average 15-20 times* [306, 307]. The value of such statements is perhaps the way they illustrate the efficiency of the enterohepatic circulation as an almost sealed recycling system which allows the most economical use of a valuable material [279].

THE FREQUENCY AND TIMING OF THE ENTEROHEPATIC CIRCULATION

It is usually stated that the bile salt pool circulates twice during the digestion of a meal. This figure is based on the intubation studies of Borgström et al. [59], who estimated that during the digestive period the duodenums of their volunteers were perfused with 4-8 g of bile salts, which is equivalent to about two pool sizes. In some subsequent studies [60] Borgström's group showed that, as little as 30 min after a meal, absorbed and re-secreted bile salts reappear in the intestinal lumen and then gradually increase in concentration. In a single experiment designed to assess the rate of recirculation, using radioactive taurocholate, they found that this enrichment reached a maximum after

---

* If, say, 18 per cent of the pool is lost per day and this is the end result of six circulations, then on average 3 per cent is lost at each circulation. This implies that on average 97 per cent of the pool is reabsorbed each time it enters the intestine. It must be emphasised that these are only average figures since it is most unlikely that the bile salt pool enters the intestine as a bolus or that the reabsorbed fraction leaves the intestine as a bolus. With this proviso it may be calculated that after 17 circulations 51 per cent or roughly half of the bile salts originally present have been excreted and therefore that 17 is the average number of times a bile salt molecule circulates.

80-90 min. If this is taken as the mean circulation time and if it is assumed that digestion of a meal takes 3-4 h, it follows that there are 2-3 circulations per meal. From these limited data it certainly seems probable that at least some of the bile salt pool enters the intestine three times per meal. It should, however, be borne in mind that these estimates derive from experiments in which healthy young men quickly drank a sweet, synthetic, liquid test meal. It is possible that the results would be different with a normal, solid, slowly chewed and incompletely digestible meal. There is clearly room for more work in this field (see Addendum at end of this chapter, page 97).

In Rhesus monkeys it has been possible to make a more direct estimate of the number of circulations daily. Using an ingenious system which allowed controlled interruptions of the enterohepatic circulation, Dowling *et al.* were able to measure both the total daily bile salt secretion and, by draining all the bile for 3 h, the total bile salt pool size. Dividing the pool into the daily secretion gave the number of circulations per day, which in four monkeys varied from 6.3 to 13.8 [154]

In the rat the number of circulations daily has been estimated by two different groups as about 12. This figure is based on the concentration of bile acids in the portal blood [489] and on the amount of infused taurocholate necessary to suppress hepatic synthesis [578]. Since the rat has no gallbladder it presumably recirculates its bile salts more frequently than normal man.

Our knowledge of the size of the bile salt pool and of the rate at which its component parts are lost and replaced derives entirely from turnover studies.

THE CONCEPT OF TURNOVER

Turnover is the term used of a homeostatically maintained pool (or of course the stock of a supermarket), a fraction of which is lost each day and replaced by new material. The turnover time is the time taken for this replacement to occur, and indicates the rate of loss of the substance. In practice the time required for complete turnover, or total replacement, cannot be measured for the following reason. If newly added material is at once mixed uniformly with old material then it will face the same risk of excretion as the old material. Consequently the more old material is diluted with new material, the slower it is excreted. This phenomenon (which perhaps explains why even a busy

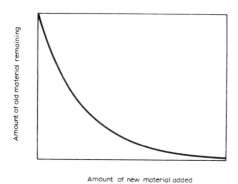

Fig. 7.2. Graph to show how the addition of new material to a turning over pool slows the rate of loss of old material.

supermarket occasionally sells bad eggs) may be represented graphically (see Fig. 7.2).

It may also be illustrated as follows. If at zero time a pool contains x g of a certain material and each day half of the pool is turned over, then on the first day $x/2$ g of our material is lost and replaced. On the second day, half of the remaining $x/2$ g is lost, that is $x/4$ g, leaving behind $x/4$ g. On the third day only $x/8$ g is lost, and so on; the amount lost is halved each day. This kind of disappearance pattern, where a constant fraction rather than a constant amount is lost per unit of time, is called exponential, and the phenomenon in question is said to follow first order kinetics. The curve that describes it has no clear end point (in theory it meets the zero line at infinity), so that the complete turnover time cannot be deduced. To overcome this, an exponential disappearance curve is normally plotted with the vertical axis on a logarithmic scale. This converts an awkward curve into a manageable straight line (Fig. 7.3).

This technique has the practical advantage of allowing the observer to draw with confidence the line that best fits his data and also to extrapolate it in either direction. The slope of the line now indicates the turnover rate, which is expressed mathematically as a decay constant K. A simpler alternative is to read off from the best-fit line the time taken for disappearance of 50 per cent of the material and to call this its half-life or $T\frac{1}{2}$. In fact $K = 0.69/T\frac{1}{2}$. K is also called the fractional turnover rate because it is the fraction of the pool turned

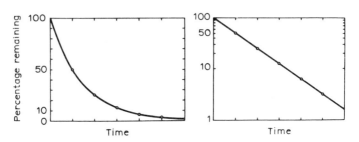

Fig. 7.3. How an exponential curve (left) is converted into a straight line (right) by using a logarithmic scale on the vertical axis.

over, that is lost or synthesised, in the time unit of K, which is usually days [313, 679].

The turnover of bile salts in the enterohepatic circulation follows first order kinetics [399, 313]. When some isotopically labelled bile salt is administered intravenously (or orally) it mixes with the endogenous pool of that bile salt and is treated by the body identically with it (such a tracer dose must be too small to expand the endogenous pool significantly, so as to avoid altering the kinetics of the pool). The rate of loss of radioactivity from the labelled bile salt fraction, that is the fall in specific activity of that bile salt, now reflects the natural turnover rate of the bile salt. This can be measured quite simply by sampling the bile repeatedly, using duodenal intubation, separating the required bile salt and measuring the radioactivity in aliquots of known mass. It is important to realise that fall in specific activity of a bile salt is not due to its excretion but to its dilution with newly synthesised non-radioactive material. However, in steady state conditions the rate of synthesis equals the rate of excretion, so that in practice the slope of the specific activity decay curve does indicate the rate of excretion of the bile salt. This is not, however, true of ileectomised patients in whom excretion is so rapid that synthesis lags behind. An example of a bile salt specific activity decay 'curve' is given in Fig. 7.4.

It must be emphasised that, no matter how near a straight line the day-by-day points of a specific activity decay curve may lie, it is most improbable that during the day bile salts are lost from the entero-hepatic circulation at anything approaching a constant rate. Firstly, it is only when a meal is eaten and the gallbladder contracts that bile salts enter the intestine and face any possibility of excretion at all. Secondly, different meals may carry quite different quantities of bile salts into the

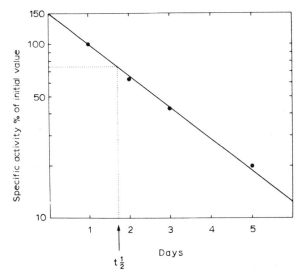

Fig. 7.4. Specific activity decay curve for taurocholate in the duodenal aspirate of a normal subject whose taurocholate pool had been labelled at zero-time with a tracer dose of sodium taurocholate-24-^{14}C. For convenience the figures for specific activity have been converted from dpm/mg to percentages of the value in the initial (24-hour) bile sample.

colon depending, for example, on their fibre content. It is therefore perhaps rather a sterile exercise to try and fit the enterohepatic circulation to a precise mathematical model [72].

To calculate from the slope of a specific activity curve the actual turnover, that is the amount of bile salt synthesised and excreted per day, it is necessary to know the pool size of that bile salt, since by definition turnover = K × pool.

DETERMINATION OF THE POOL SIZE OF A BILE SALT

The only accurate way of determining the pool size under physiological conditions is by the technique of isotope dilution. The principle of this is to measure the specific activity of the required bile salt, isolated from the bile immediately after it has mixed with a known amount of radioactivity. If a total of A dpm (disintegrations per minute) are administered, and the zero-time specific activity is B dpm/mg, then the size of the repleted pool (Fig. 7.1) in mg is A/B.

TABLE 7.1. *Published values for b*

Reference	Method	Number of subjects	Diet	Total bile acid synthesis (by summation) (mg/day)	Total acid p (by summ (g)
Danielsson et al. (1963)	Isotope dilution (cholic acid-^{3}H and chenodeoxycholic acid-^{14}C)	2 (age and sex unspecified)	40% calories as butter fat	535 (490, 580)	—
Danzinger et al. (1971a)	Isotope dilution (chenodeoxycholic acid-^{3}H and -^{2}H)	2 (age and sex unspecified)	Unspecified	—	—
Hellström (1965)	Isotope dilution (cholic acid-^{14}C)	3 (F aged 20-22)	Low cholesterol formula diet	—	2.82 (1.91-3
Hellström & Lindstedt (1966)	Isotope dilution (cholic acid-^{14}C)	9 (6 F aged 19-40, 3 M aged 25-37)	40% calories as butter fat 40% calories as corn oil	— —	3.2C (1.87-5 3.46 (2.00-5
Kottke (1969)	Isotope dilution (cholic acid-^{14}C and chenodeoxy-cholic acid-^{3}H)	2 (age and sex unspecified)	Low fat, low cholesterol	451 (one subject)	—
Lindstedt (1957a)	Isotope dilution (Cholic acid-24-^{14}C)	8 (male medical students)	Free	—	3.5 (1.88-4
Lindstedt et al. (1965)	Isotope dilution (cholic acid-^{14}C)	2 (F 61, M 28) 4 (2 F 20 and 21, 2 M 19, 20) Ditto	Normal Corn oil enriched Coconut oil enriched	— — —	— — —
Vlahcevic et al. (1970a)	Isotope dilution (cholic acid-^{14}C)	9 (M aged 32-76; hospital patients)	2,500 calories	—	2.3 (1.70-
Vlahcevic et al. (1971)	Isotope dilution (cholic acid-^{14}C and chenodeoxy-cholic acid-^{14}C)	10 (M 41-72, hospital patients)	2,500 calories	495 (265-875)	2.2 (1.68-2
Meihoff & Kern (1968)	Isotope excretion (cholic acid-^{14}C)	7 (4 M, 3 F, young adults)	Free	—	—
Stanley & Nemchausky (1967)	Isotope excretion (cholic acid-^{14}C)	16 (half male, aged 4-51)	Standard but normal	—	—

* Value for pool size obtained indirectly by chemical ratios of bile salts in bile.
† Calculated by the author from data given in the reference cited.

in normal man (means and ranges)

	Cholate			Chenodeoxycholate		Deoxycholate
size g)	Turnover (mg/day)	Half-life (days)	Pool size (g)	Turnover (mg/day)	Half-life (days)	Pool size (g)
82 1.19)	195 (190, 200)	3.0 (2.0, 4.0)	2.47 (2.42, 2.52)	340 (290, 390)	5.1 (4.3, 6.0)	—
—	—	—	1.10 (1.05, 1.15)	145 (75, 215)	7.0† (3.4, 10.6)	—
60 1.90)	355 (265-410)	3.3 (2.2-5.0)	0.94*† (0.48-1.30)	—	—	0.28*† (0.19-0.35)
12 2.02)	295 (80-450)	3.2 (1.4-6.5)	1.23*† (0.63-2.16)	—	—	0.95*† (0.15-1.80)
29 2.08)	314 (140-480)	3.2 (1.5-6.5)	1.27*† (0.71-2.51)	—	—	0.94*† (0.28-2.57)
—	273 (263, 283)	—	—	188 (one subject)	—	—
38 2.29)	360 (210-690)	2.8 (1.2-4.2)	1.45* (0.79-1.88)	—	—	0.77* (0.51-1.10)
34 1.24)	135 (90, 180)	4.1 (3.3, 5.0)	—	—	—	—
24 1.76)	195 (130-240)	4.5 (2.7-5.9)	—	—	—	—
77 0.99)	148 (110-210)	3.9 (2.5-5.0)	—	—	—	—
8 1.78)	358 (140-610)	2.8 (1.3-6.2)	0.83*	—	—	0.31* (0.05-0.62)
04 1.36)	333 (160-629)	2.2† (1.3-5.2)	0.81 (0.64-1.15)	162 (75-247)	3.1† (1.9-7.1)	0.38* (0.01-0.72)
	—	6.2† (3.3-10.5)	—	—	—	—
	—	7.4 ± S.E. 0.97	—	—	—	—

The figure *A/B* represents the number of times the radioactive bolus was diluted as it mixed with the endogenous pool.

Unfortunately, several enterohepatic cycles are probably necessary for thorough mixing of exogenous isotope with endogenous pool, so that zero-time specific activity cannot be measured directly. Some workers have assumed that they obtained an adequate approximation of zero-time specific activity by aspirating the duodenal contents with the help of injected cholecystokinin 3 h after intravenous injection of the isotope and then mixing it *in vitro* before taking an aliquot for analysis [1]. However, this assumption cannot be accepted without careful validation. This limitation is overcome by measuring specific activity in serial bile samples obtained over the course of several days, starting 24 h after the isotope was administered, and extrapolating the decay curve back to zero-time. The figure so obtained is used to calculate isotope dilution. Published figures for the pool sizes of cholic and chenodeoxycholic acids measured in this way are shown in Table 7.1. Once the pool size of one bile acid has been measured, that of the others can be calculated by measuring chemically the ratios between the main bile acid fractions. Simple addition gives the total bile salt pool.

The effective bile salt pool size can be estimated semi-quantitatively by measuring the total bile salt concentration in post-prandial duodenal contents [313]. However, this figure is affected by other factors besides the pool size, such as the rate of gallbladder emptying and the extent of dilution of bile with other digestive juices.

OTHER METHODS FOR MEASURING HALF-LIFE AND TURNOVER RATE OF BILE ACIDS

Conceptually, the simplest way of measuring bile acid turnover is *chemical estimation of the faecal bile acids.* However, this is technically very complex and has not been widely practised. Moreover this technique gives no information on the pool size or half-life of bile salts. A further difficulty is the fact that figures for synthesis rate obtained in this way are often lower than those obtained by bile acid specific activity measurements. This discrepancy has not been explained. There is good evidence that the steroid nucleus of cholesterol is degraded during intestinal passage but this has not been shown for bile acids [247]. Loss in the urine accounts for only 4 per cent of bile acid excretion in man [120] (unlike rabbits who excrete 10 per cent of their bile acids in the urine [292]). The chemical 'balance' method is discussed in detail by Hofmann and his colleagues [313].

The *isotope excretion method* depends on the simple estimation of faecal radioactivity against an internal marker such as chromium sesquioxide after administration of a known amount of radioactive bile acid by mouth. It gives no information other than the half-life or decay constant K, but has been useful in demonstrating bile acid malabsorption [313, 426, 622].

The *isotope derivative method* (or isotope balance method) is the measurement of bile acid radioactivity in the stool after intravenous administration of labelled cholesterol. Division of this measurement by the serum cholesterol specific activity gives the mass of faecal bile acids. Rather complex stool extraction, much time and a lot of radioactivity are required, and the method has not become popular [313]. It has been used to show the effects of dietary fats, of cholestyramine and of ileal bypass on bile acid excretion [447-449].

THE KINETICS OF BILE SALT TURNOVER IN NORMAL MAN

Figures obtained by these various methods in subjects on different diets are given in Tables 7.1 and 7.2. Certain comments may be made about these data.

(1) There is much individual variation. This necessitates using subjects as their own controls as far as possible when studying the effect of a diet or other regime.

(2) If the average half-life of cholic acid is taken as three days this agrees well with the calculation that on average a bile salt molecule circulates 17 times, on the assumption that there are six circulations per day.

(3) The half-life of cholic acid is found to be twice as long by the isotope excretion method as by the isotope dilution method. The basis of this anomaly has not been studied, but some delay due to colonic transit is to be expected between loss of cholic acid from the bile and its appearance in the stool. Also, some lost 'cholic' acid continues to circulate in the form of deoxycholate.

(4) Chenodeoxycholate is turned over somewhat more slowly than cholate. This has also been noted in hypercholesterolaemic

TABLE 7.2. *Published values for faecal excretion of bile acids in normal man*

Reference	Method	Number of subjects	Diet	Total bile acid excretion (mg/day)
Moore et al. (1968)	Isotope derivative method	5 (M, 20-29)	Butter-containing	473 ± S.E.19
			Safflower oil-containing	564 ± S.E.36
Avigan & Steinberg (1965)	Isotope derivative method	6 (age and sex unspecified)	Liquid formula diet (60% calories as fat) (a) Coconut oil (b) Corn/safflower oil	(a) 1,030 (240-2,200) (b) 840 (100-2,320)
Wilson & Lindsey (1965)	Isotope derivative method	2 (M, 31 and 23)	Liquid formula diet (a) High cholesterol (b) Low cholesterol	(a) 1030, 280 (b) 830, 230
Ali et al. (1966a)	Chemical estimation	3 (M, middle-aged)	Fat-free	410 (130-649)
Miettinen et al. (1967)	Chemical estimation	19 (10 M, 9 F; hospital patients aged about 30-50)	Normal, constant	220 ± S.E.16
Connor et al. (1969)	Chemical estimation	6 (M, 36-44)	Liquid formula diet (a) Cocoa-butter (b) Corn oil	(a) 271 (88-2070) (b) 426 (183-1321)

patients [367, 707]. The chenodeoxycholate half-life is generally about 50 per cent longer than the cholate half-life. Whether this is due to readier absorption or greater resistance to bacterial attack is unknown. Curiously, the opposite pattern has been noted in cirrhotic patients [700] and in rodents [29].

(5) It is noteworthy that the deoxycholate and lithocholate pools have never been measured directly, and that their turnover rates have never been measured at all.

(6) With isotope dilution studies, at least on middle-aged subjects, it is essential to state whether the gallbladder is functional and

TABLE 7.3. *The kinetics of taurocholate and glycocholate in man (isotope dilution studies)*

Reference	Number of subjects	Diet	Taurocholate			Glycocholate		
			Half-life (days)	Pool size (g)	Turnover (mg/day)	Half-life (days)	Pool size (g)	Turnover (mg/day)
Austad et al. (1967)	2 (male students)	Free	2.1 (1.9, 2.3)	0.33 (0.30, 0.36)	108 (107, 110)	—	—	—
Heaton et al. (1968)	6 (male 22-25)	Free	1.9 (1.4-2.2)	0.38 (0.27-0.63)	144 (84-237)	—	—	—
	3 (male 22-25)	Free	—	—	—	1.38 (1.25-1.55)	1.16 (0.73-1.60)	533 (407-715)
Pomare & Heaton (1971)	6 (female 41-58)	Free	1.5 (0.9-2.6)	0.30 (0.14-0.66)	142 (74-218)	—	—	—

normal. To date, this has only been done in the studies of Vlahcevic *et al.* [679, 684].

The isotope dilution technique has been used to study the turnover of *taurocholate* and *glycocholate* and the data obtained are given in Table 7.3. It will be noted that the half-lives of these conjugated bile salts are shorter than those of free cholate. In the case of taurocholate this is because its specific activity declines for another reason besides dehydroxylation and excretion, namely bacterial deconjugation followed by absorption of labelled cholate and recirculation after hepatic conjugation with glycine in preference to taurine. With glycocholate this mechanism can play little part, but so few subjects have been studied that the low figure for $T\frac{1}{2}$ may be fortuitous. It must, however, be admitted that different conjugated bile salts may well show different kinetics—the problem has simply not been explored.

Studies of taurocholate turnover can usefully be combined with analysis of recirculated metabolites of taurocholate [214, 278]. We have used this technique to demonstrate subnormal dehydroxylation of bile salts in subjects without a colon [454], and increased dehydroxylation in subjects without a gallbladder [517].

KINETICS OF BILE SALTS IN OTHER SPECIES

Bile salt kinetics have been studied in the rat [29, 251, 256, 258, 403, 404, 525, 629], mouse [29], hamster [29], gerbil [29], rabbit [292, 293], dog [210, 513, 706] and Rhesus monkey [154]. These investigations have yielded important information regarding the effects of diet, hormones and bacteria, and the role of the ileum and the gallbladder. Recent discussions of these studies are to be found in the reviews of Weiner & Lack [691] and of Danielsson & Tchen [125]. The results of these studies should not be applied too closely to man because, for example, the rat has no gallbladder and the rat and rabbit eat their faeces.

HOMEOSTASIS: THE CONTROL OF BILE SALT SYNTHESIS

The liver has a great reserve capacity for bile salt production and normally its synthetic activity is held in check. This is best shown by the effects of a biliary fistula. When a rat's common bile duct is cannulated there is in the first 6-12 h a high excretion of bile salts as the circulating pool is washed out [178, 179, 506]. For the next 12 h or so there is a low rate of excretion which equals the normal synthetic rate, but thereafter the rate rises rapidly so that after 48 h it reaches a plateau at a value 10-20 times the basal rate. The latter presumably indicates maximal hepatic synthesis; it continues even when the liver is removed and perfused outside the animal [506]. In man, too, biliary drainage causes a marked rise in bile salt synthesis. In nine patients with complete external bile fistulas the total synthesis rate averaged 3.3 g/day (cholate 2.1 g, chenodeoxycholate 1.2 g) [94]. Since the normal synthesis rate is probably about 500 mg/day (see Table 7.1), this represents a six- to sevenfold increase. Similarly the Rhesus monkey can increase its synthesis rate tenfold [154].

Besides biliary drainage there are two other ways in which the enterohepatic circulation can be interrupted. These are resection of the ileum and oral administration of a bile salt-sequestrating agent, such as cholestyramine. Both these measures result in a four- to eightfold increase in bile salt excretion and therefore in bile salt synthesis [248, 273, 448, 459, 709]. This indicates that the factor (or factors) controlling bile salt synthesis is in some way related to the entero-hepatic circulation. It has been shown in Rhesus monkeys that the liver is very responsive to minor alterations of the enterohepatic circulation. Diversion of as little as 10 per cent of the animal's bile flow is detected and compensated for by increased synthesis of bile salts [154].

The obvious interpretation of these facts is that the controlling factor is bile salts themselves. It is an attractive idea that bile salts should exert negative feedback on their own synthesis and it has a good deal of experimental support. The best evidence comes from studies in which infusing bile salts into the duodenum of rats prevented the usual rise in hepatic synthesis produced by biliary drainage. This phenome-non was first demonstrated with taurochenodeoxycholate [36], and there is some evidence that this di-hydroxy bile salt is a more potent inhibitor than taurocholate [382]. However, it has been shown that taurocholate is an efficient inhibitor if given in doses large enough to match the rapid circulation of the rat's bile salt pool [578]. It is likely that certain bile acids are more inhibitory than others. *In vitro*, free bile acids are more potent than conjugates, and di-hydroxy more potent than tri-hydroxy, at inhibiting mitochondrial oxidation of the first intermediate compounds in the two pathways of bile acid synthesis,

7α-hydroxy cholesterol and 26-hydroxy cholesterol [137]. However, this could be an artefact of *in vitro* toxicity [241]. In support of bile acid-bile acid negative feedback is the report that feeding taurocholate to man causes a flattening out of the serum cholesterol specific activity decay curve [249]. Further, it has been demonstrated that feeding chenodeoxycholate causes a virtual disappearance of cholate and deoxycholate from the bile salt pool [656], in other words an almost complete cessation of cholic acid synthesis. Recently, Low-Beer *et al.* [411a] have produced suggestive evidence for a specific effect of deoxycholate in suppressing synthesis of chenodeoxycholate.

It is not yet clear whether this controlling effect is only upon bile acid synthesis or whether it is also upon cholesterol synthesis. Certainly one rate-controlled step is 7α-hydroxylation of cholesterol, the first step up in bile acid synthesis, [123, 579]. However, interrupting the enterohepatic circulation causes a marked increase in cholesterol synthesis [462] and this seems to precede the increase in bile acid synthesis by about 8 h [122]. Thus it may be argued that the primary effect is on cholesterol synthesis, probably at the stage of mevalonic acid synthesis from β-hydroxy-β-methylglutaryl CoA [149], and that changes in bile acid synthesis follow secondarily [112].

Recently Dietschy & Wilson have advanced the theory that the factor controlling bile salt synthesis is not reabsorbed bile salts in the portal blood but cholesterol going from the intestine in the lymph and thence in the arterial blood [149]. They argue that, if control is exerted primarily on cholesterol synthesis, then the controlling factor should be the same as that for cholesterol synthesis (which they have convincingly shown to be chylomicron cholesterol [149]). They would explain the inhibitory effects of bile salt feeding noted above by saying that there was expansion of the bile salt pool and hence increased cholesterol absorption. However this theory lacks evidence. In dogs and rats, feeding cholesterol results in increased, not decreased, bile salt synthesis [2, 701], while in man there is probably no effect [287, 527, 702].

THE EFFECTS OF INTERRUPTION OF THE ENTEROHEPATIC CIRCULATION

It has been noted above that any manoeuvre which interrupts the enterohepatic circulation causes a marked increase in bile acid synthesis by the liver. When the interruption is slight it is compensated for by this increased synthesis. In the Rhesus monkey the limit is reached at 20 per cent interruption [154]. At this point total daily bile salt secretion is well maintained, though at the price of a 10-fold increase in synthesis. At 33 per cent interruption there is a marked reduction in bile salt secretion, to less than 60 per cent of normal. This very limited capacity of the liver to compensate is perhaps most easily understood by comparing the amount of bile salt which perfuses the human intestine on a normal day when a 3 g pool circulates six times, namely 18 g, with the maximum synthetic capacity of the liver, namely 3.3 g/day. With these figures in mind it is easy to understand why disease or resection of the ileum leads to bile salt deficiency (see Chapter 10).

Chronic interruption of the enterohepatic circulation involves a great increase in cholesterol turnover and usually a fall in serum cholesterol. Ileal bypass and cholestyramine are both used in the treatment of hypercholesterolaemia (see Chapters 10 and 15).

Acute interruption of the enterohepatic circulation causes a fall in the bile salt/cholesterol and lecithin/cholesterol ratios in the bile [475, 662], such that the bile is supersaturated with cholesterol [155, 475]. This phenomenon may be relevant to the problem of gallstone formation (see Chapter 12). When an interruption is prolonged, at least in Rhesus monkeys, the cholesterol-solubilising capacity of the bile increases due to an enhanced secretion of phospholipid, but the bile remains saturated with cholesterol [155].

Addendum to page 84

Since this chapter was written, workers at the Mayo clinic, using liquid feeds and an intubation technique which allows estimation of total daily bile salt secretion, have shown that the frequency of enterohepatic cycling is proportional to the size of meals. On a diet supplying 40 kcal./kg/day, the daily number of cycles in five subjects varied from 5 to 13 with a mean of 9 [72a].

8 The Functions of Bile Salts

The functions of bile salts may be summarised under four headings:

Bile secretion: Bile salts promote excretion of water, lecithin, cholesterol and pigment.

Lipid digestion-absorption: Bile salts help to emulsify fat; assist pancreatic lipolysis; solubilise products of lipolysis together with other insoluble lipids by forming mixed micelles; possibly stimulate intracellular re-esterification of fatty acids and formation of chylomicrons.

Small intestinal function: Bile salts release hormones and perhaps enterokinase; control cholesterol synthesis by mucosa; possibly cleanse mucosa and prevent bacterial growth.

Colonic function: Bile salts possibly promote motility and prevent undue dehydration of faeces.

BILE SALTS AND THE SECRETION OF BILE

Bile salts are by far the most abundant of the organic solids in bile, being present in hepatic bile in a concentration of about 1800 mg per cent (36 mM) [81]. By contrast, the other three major organic solids in bile are present in the following average concentrations: lecithin 710 mg per cent, cholesterol 130 mg per cent, bilirubin 92 mg per cent. The electrolytes sodium, potassium, calcium, magnesium, and chloride are present in concentrations similar to those in blood, but bicarbonate is rather higher at 27-55 mM [662].

The sheer abundance of bile salts makes it likely that they play an important role in the process of bile secretion. Indeed, since the work of Sperber [617, 618] it is standard teaching [696] that the prime motive force in the formation of bile by the hepatocyte is the active transport of bile salts across the canalicular membrane. This theory invokes osmotic attraction by the transported bile acids and their associated cations as the cause of passive transfer of water and electrolytes into the canalicular lumen. Support for this idea comes from the well-known superiority of dehydrocholate (the tri-keto analogue of cholate, sold commercially as Decholin) over natural bile salts as a choleretic agent, since dehydrocholate does not form micelles and therefore mole for mole exerts a higher osmotic force [618]. (On passage through the liver of the rat some dehydrocholate is metabolised to other substances including cholic acid but their ability to form micelles is still minimal [268].) Furthermore when taurocholate is infused intravenously into dogs at different rates there is a linear correlation between the rate of infusion and the bile flow rate [695]. In man acute interruption of the enterohepatic circulation of bile salts by diversion of bile flow causes the rate of bile secretion to fall by about half [662].

Recently the supremacy of bile salts in bile secretion has been challenged by the discovery that a substantial fraction of canalicular bile secretion is independent of bile salts [180]. Indeed, in the isolated rat liver this fraction seems to be the main source of bile secretion pressure, while in the rabbit and hamster it may account for 60 per cent of the total bile flow [180, 360]. Its driving force is probably active transport of sodium [180] and it may be involved in the choleretic response to a variety of agents, including hydrocortisone [420] and phenobarbitone [43, 363]. (Recent work, however, strongly suggests that phenobarbitone increases bile salt secretion [3, 530] and even bile salt synthesis [530].)

The relative importance of these two mechanisms for bile secretion varies in different species [68, 362]. Where there is a low resting flow rate, that is a small bile salt independent fraction, as in the dog, there is also a marked choleretic response to bile salts. The rat and rabbit have a high resting flow of dilute bile and a much smaller response to bile salts [362]. The position in man is unknown.

For completeness it should be added that a third component of bile secretion exists in the form of a bicarbonate-rich fraction, probably secreted by the ducts under the influence of secretin [695], vagal stimulation and possibly other hormones [71, 72].

INFLUENCE OF BILE SALTS ON BILIARY LECITHIN
AND CHOLESTEROL

Recently much evidence has accumulated to suggest that the secretion of both these lipids into bile is largely dependent on bile salt secretion. This is particularly true of lecithin, the main biliary phospholipid. When the enterohepatic circulation is interrupted acutely the biliary secretion of lecithin falls almost as rapidly as that of bile salts [476, 662], and it increases rapidly when bile salts are re-fed [476, 31], infused into the portal vein [277] or added to the perfusate of an isolated liver [636, 638]. All this suggests either that lecithin is passively 'washed' into the bile in bile salt micelles or that bile salts increase the synthesis of lecithin. Studies of the incorporation of labelled precursors into bile lecithin have shown that the synthesis of lecithin is in fact increased by bile salts [22, 477]. The fact that an artificial bile salt glycodehydrocholate, which does not form micelles, does not increase phospholipid secretion, has been taken as evidence that phospholipid is incorporated into micelles prior to its secretion [712]. However, it is not known how glycodehydrocholate affects phospholipid synthesis.

Two groups of workers have shown a direct correlation between bile salt pool size and phospholipid secretion [476, 637]. Since lecithin is as important as bile salts in maintaining cholesterol in solution in the bile, it is clear that the problem of cholesterol solubility and therefore of gallstone formation is very closely related to the size of the circulating bile salt pool and the factors affecting it (see Chapter 12).

The influence of bile salts on cholesterol secretion is less well understood. There is no doubt that in man acute interruption of the enterohepatic circulation causes a fall in cholesterol secretion [476, 662]. However, this fall is less than the fall in bile salt and lecithin secretion. Moreover, feeding and withdrawing bile salts has relatively little immediate effect on cholesterol secretion [31]. This suggests either that biliary cholesterol excretion is largely independent of the availability of bile salts, or that there is a delayed response to changes in the amount of bile salts passing through the liver. By contrast, with the isolated perfused rat liver, altering the rate of bile salt in fusion causes changes in bile cholesterol output which are as prompt and as large as changes in lecithin secretion, suggesting that all three components are secreted together in the form of micellar aggregates [269]. Whether this difference is due to genuine species variation or merely to different experimental techniques is unclear.

The close association between the secretion of bile salts and that of phospholipid and cholesterol has led to speculations that bile salts either leach out these lipids on their way through the canalicular membrane or even cause the membrane to bud off into the canalicular lumen in the form of small vesicles [64].

INFLUENCE OF BILE SALTS ON BILE PIGMENT EXCRETION

It is debatable whether or not bile salts and bile pigment share a common biliary transport system [338]. It is hard to demonstrate competition experimentally and even harder to believe it occurs physiologically. On the contrary, there is evidence from hamster studies that bile salt transport enhances bilirubin transport [359], perhaps because bilirubin is included in bile salt-lipid micelles [365, 67].

It seems likely that bile salt secretion similarly aids the excretion of 'detoxicated' hormones and drugs.

BILE SALTS AND LIPID ABSORPTION

The importance of bile salts in fat absorption is evidenced by the steatorrhoea that follows bile diversion, ileal disorders and administration of cholestyramine. However, even complete diversion of bile allows at least 50 per cent of the dietary fat to be absorbed, showing that bile salts merely assist and accelerate the absorption of triglycerides. On the other hand, the absorption of cholesterol, fat-soluble vitamins and other insoluble lipids is almost totally dependent on bile and is virtually abolished by bile diversion. Bile salts are probably not directly involved in the digestion or absorption of carbohydrates and proteins [307]. However, indirect influences may exist since, according to recent studies, infusion of bile salts into the duodenum stimulates the secretion of enzyme-rich pancreatic juice [193, 710]. In addition, there is *in vitro* evidence that bile salts release enterokinase (the activator of trypsinogen) from the small bowel brush border [260] (although the physiological significance of this phenomenon has been questioned [478]) and that they increase mucosal permeability to ionised materials [219], and alter the electrical properties of the mucosa [185].

EMULSIFICATION

It used to be thought that the main digestive role of bile salts was to emulsify dietary fat. In fact bile salts are poor emulsifiers unless accompanied by a polar lipid (or, more accurately, a swelling amphiphile), such as lecithin or monoglyceride [200]. Fat leaves the stomach as a coarse emulsion. This emulsion is probably made finer through the surface tension-lowering action of, initially, bile salts and lecithin and later of bile salts and monoglycerides. Lysolecithin, released by partial hydrolysis of lecithin, is also an effective emulsifier. It has been questioned whether formation of a fine emulsion is an important phase in fat digestion because lipolysis is an explosively rapid process and its products are immediately taken up into micellar solution [307].

PANCREATIC LIPOLYSIS

The function of pancreatic lipase is a chemical one, namely to split by hydrolysis the 1- or α-ester bonds of triglycerides, and so release 2-monoglycerides and fatty acids [307]. This chemical process results in major changes in the physical state of intraluminal fat. Hofmann has suggested that the essential role of lipase is 'to transform triglyceride, which is not penetrated by water, into lipolytic products which together form a dispersible, liquid crystalline phase' [308]. If such a phase does form on the surface of the emulsion particle it is certainly transitory, being immediately dispersed by bile salts into micelles. The action of lipase is assisted by bile salts in five ways:

(1) By aiding emulsification bile salts increase the surface area of the oil-water interface at which lipase works.
(2) Bile salts 'activate' lipase, perhaps by inducing a configurational change in the enzyme molecule [141].
(3) Bile salts reduce the pH optimum of lipase [55].
(4) In combining with released 2-monoglyceride and fatty acid bile salts displace lipase to a new interface [160].
(5) Incorporation of fatty acids into micelles increases their ionisation and so renders them less available for re-esterification by lipase working 'in reverse'; thus lipolysis is driven to completion [304].

In spite of all this it has been difficult [100] or impossible [364, 520] to demonstrate impaired lipolysis in bile-diverted animals and it is doubtful if this is the rate-limiting step in fat absorption in the absence of bile [134].

MICELLAR SOLUBILISATION

Ultra-centrifugation of the contents of the upper small intestine after a meal show it to consist of a large aqueous phase, a small oil phase and a sediment. The oil phase contains most of the triglyceride and diglyceride, together with some monoglyceride and unionised fatty acid. The aqueous phase contains most of the fatty acid, variable amounts of monoglyceride and very little higher glycerides, as well of course as the bile salts. In the aqueous phase the lipids are believed to be held in micellar solution, the micelles consisting mainly of bile salt, monoglyceride and partly ionised fatty acids or soaps, as explained in Chapter 3. The importance of the micellar phase lies presumably in the very small size of the micelles which enables them to penetrate between intestinal microvilli and in general increases the chances of contact between lipid and absorptive membrane. This is illustrated in Fig. 8.1. This figure does not show the insoluble lipids, cholesterol and fat-soluble vitamins, which are partitioned between the three phases.

It seems likely that under normal conditions the micellar phase is the final common pathway for the absorption of all lipids. Certainly fatty acids, monoglycerides and cholesterol are efficiently taken up by segments of jejunum perfused with micellar solutions [60, 588], and in vitro the intestine takes up monoglyceride and fatty acid twice as rapidly from a micellar solution as from a suspension [341]. Moreover in human perfusion studies the rate of fat absorption was proportional to the micellar fatty acid concentration and to the total bile salt concentration [694]. In spite of this, there is good evidence from studies in rats that fatty acid absorption can proceed as efficiently from an emulsion as from a micellar solution [263, 450, 589], or nearly so [300]. In man, too, it has been suggested that the role of micelles in fatty acid absorption has been overemphasised, since patients with bile drainage may have negligible micellar fatty acid in their intestinal aspirate and yet have normal fat absorption morphologically and only mild steatorrhoea [519, 520]. Probably, of the two main end products of pancreatic lipolysis it is only monoglycerides which are very dependent for their absorption on solubilisation in bile salt micelles. In the absence of bile, fatty acids are quite well absorbed from emulsion

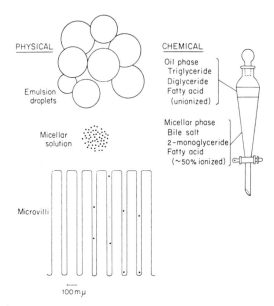

Fig. 8.1. Diagram to show the physical and chemical states of lipids in intestinal contents during fat digestion and absorption. The oil and micellar phases are in equilibrium with each other, and presumably with the little-studied sediment. The emulsion droplets, micelles (shown as black dots) and microvilli are drawn approximately to scale (from Hofmann [304]).

droplets by simple molecular diffusion [263, 451], but the concentration of monoglycerides in the intestinal lumen tends to remain high [364].

It has recently been suggested that the function of the mixed micelle in fatty acid absorption is simply to maintain a high concentration of fatty acid in the 200μ thick 'unstirred' water layer immediately adjacent to the absorptive membrane [544]. Schultz & Strecker, however, consider it more likely that the micelle enters the brush border and breaks up within it [572].

THE MUCOSAL PHASE OF FAT ABSORPTION

The sequence of events at the brush order is controversial. One group of workers found that rat jejunum incubated in a micellar solution took up taurodeoxycholate and oleic acid in exactly equimolar amounts and suggested that the entire mixed micelle diffuses into the cell [230]. However, other investigators using a similar technique came to the opposite conclusion [661]. If bile salts are absorbed (or adsorbed) in this way in the jejunum they must be returned to the lumen. Evidence for such a return has been presented [440]. In any case, it seems certain that by some means or other, bile salts accelerate fatty acid uptake by the intestine [102, 341, 510].

Having reached the interior of the mucosal cell, fatty acids are rapidly esterified to re-form triglycerides and then incorporated into chylomicrons. Another unsettled question is whether conjugated bile salts stimulate this re-esterification process. Since such an effect was first reported by Dawson & Isselbacher in 1960 [135] it has been confirmed [364], denied [450], confirmed again [100, 355], denied again [511] and confirmed yet again [102, 536].

It is difficult to reconcile this intracellular role of bile salts with the absence of significant bile salt absorption in the jejunum (pages 75-78). The most quoted evidence for such a role is the undoubted fact that during digestion the mucosa of the bile fistula animal contains reduced concentrations of di- and triglyceride and an excess of fatty acid [100, 355, 364, 536]. However, as Hofmann has pointed out [307], this may merely reflect the difficulty that the bile fistula animal has in solubilising and absorbing monoglyceride. Starved of monoglyceride, the cell would be deprived of its main pathway of triglyceride re-synthesis (2-monoglyceride plus two fatty acid molecules → triglyceride [350]). At the same time, the still freely entering fatty acids would not be utilised quickly enough by the second pathway of triglyceride synthesis (α-glycerophosphate plus three fatty acid molecules → triglyceride) to prevent fatty acid accumulating in the cell. This explanation has been supported by the finding that bile fistula rats differ from normal animals in that when given triolein they absorb it preferentially as fatty acid rather than as monoglyceride [451]. However, the case has been re-opened by the recent *in vitro* finding [231] that bile salts do stimulate the enzymes of the monoglyceride pathway, while having no effect on the glycerophosphate pathway. Absence of this stimulation would account for the reduced triglyceride synthesis of the bile-depleted animal and also provide an additional explanation for its monoglyceride malabsorption, namely reduced clearance of monoglyceride from the absorptive cell resulting in loss of the concentration gradient from lumen to cell.

Recently, evidence has been presented for another intracellular role of bile salts—the stimulation of triglyceride synthesis from phospholipids in jejunal mucosa [667].

One point on which there does appear to be general agreement is that in the absence of bile the route of fat absorption is altered, so that very few chylomicrons enter the lymph and more fatty acids are carried in the portal vein [136]. This has been shown in man using radioactive fatty acids [50].

Obviously the relationship between bile and fat absorption is complex. However, it does at least seem certain that it is only the bile salt fraction of bile which is important, since the absorption defects of a bile fistula animal are completely corrected by the oral administration of bile salts [136]. A synthetic detergent such as Tween 80 is also moderately effective [136]. Bile salts may assist fat digestion and absorption in other more indirect ways as well as through their detergent properties. Bile diversion leads for some reason to delayed gastric emptying [355, 364] and, as already noted, bile salts may be necessary for optimal stimulation of pancreatic secretion [193, 710].

A useful review of bile salts and fat absorption has appeared recently [587].

BILE SALTS AND THE ABSORPTION OF FAT-SOLUBLE VITAMINS

There is virtually no absorption of vitamins A, D, E and K in bile-diverted animals [307], while in patients with complete biliary obstruction there is little or no recovery of orally administered radioactive vitamins from a cannula in the thoracic duct [195]. Thus these water-insoluble vitamins are almost completely dependent on bile for their absorption. Bile salts are undoubtedly the vital factor, since feeding them to a bile fistula animal corrects its absorption defect [307], while in rats feeding cholestyramine interferes with vitamin D absorption [660]. Similarly, in man the rise in serum vitamin A after an oral load is much reduced if a large dose of cholestyramine is given at the same time [24, 407]. Since fat-soluble vitamins are water-insoluble polar lipids (non-swelling amphiphiles) they require incorporation into mixed micelles for their solubilisation and absorption (see page 29). Probably for this reason their absorption is promoted by the ingestion of triglyceride and reduced by the ingestion of mineral oil [307]. In addition, fatty acid is needed to make the chylomicrons in which the vitamin is transported out of the mucosa, and this explains why in rats, vitamin D is absorbed better from a mixed micellar solution than from pure bile salt micelles [659].

In vitro the absorption of vitamin D is enhanced by taurocholate but not by taurochenodeoxycholate or taurodeoxycholate [555]. The physiological significance of this phenomenon is uncertain.

To be absorbed, the main dietary form of vitamin A, β-carotene, must be split enzymatically by the intestinal mucosa to release retinol ester. *In vitro*, bile salts and especially the taurine conjugates stimulate the uptake and cleavage of β-carotene [490].

BILE SALTS AND CHOLESTEROL ABSORPTION

Cholesterol resembles the fat-soluble vitamins in being insoluble in water, and in needing mixed micelles for its solubilisation (see Chapter 3). This makes it entirely dependent upon bile salts for its transport to the brush border. If presented to the mucosa in a micellar solution it is rapidly absorbed [588, 640]. However, after a test meal [56], or in intestinal perfusion studies [588], it is absorbed less rapidly than monoglycerides and fatty acids. Since these are as necessary as bile salts for the formation of mixed micelles, cholesterol is never completely absorbed. The residue mixes with the sediment phase of intestinal contents [588]. It is likely that in the normally feeding animal most of the cholesterol is present in the sediment, but this does not mean it cannot be made available for absorption [418]. As with fat-soluble vitamins, absorption of cholesterol is increased by feeding fat [61, 665], is decreased by feeding cholestyramine [448] and is virtually abolished by bile diversion [591]. In rats the absorption of cholesterol from a test meal was proportional to the amount of bile salts added to the test meal [209].

It is likely that bile salts influence the mucosal stage of cholesterol absorption since, in the absence of bile, cholesterol synthesised locally in the intestinal wall is not delivered to the lymph [703]. This effect may be on either esterification of cholesterol or the subsequent transfer of chylomicrons into the lymph [149].

In a study in rats, taurochenodeoxycholate was more effective than the other bile salts tested at stimulating cholesterol absorption, including its esterification by the mucosa [209].

A cholesterol esterase is secreted in the pancreatic juice and its activity is dependent on bile salts, which also protect the enzyme from inactivation by chymotrypsin [665]. However, these effects may not be physiologically important since normally only free cholesterol enters the intestine in the diet and in the bile [307].

Apparently, absorption of *other sterols* such as plant sterols is also (to the small extent that it occurs) dependent upon micellar solubilisation and therefore upon bile salts [58, 640].

BILE SALTS AND THE CONTROL OF CHOLESTEROL SYNTHESIS BY INTESTINE AND LIVER

It has recently been discovered that the gastro-intestinal tract is an important source of serum cholesterol [398] and that the most active area of synthesis is the terminal ileum. In both rat [146] and man [147] the terminal ileum is three or four times more active in this respect than the next most active area, the duodenum. Intestinal cholesterol synthesis is greatly enhanced by bile diversion [146, 147] but returns to normal with infusion of bile salts into the intestine [146]. These and other experiments [146] prove that normally bile salts exert a controlling effect on intestinal cholesterol synthesis. This is important because, gram for gram, the human intestine can probably synthesise cholesterol as fast as the liver [149].

Until recently it was widely believed that cholesterol synthesis by the liver is controlled by bile acids in the enterohepatic circulation. The evidence for bile acid-cholesterol feedback, obtained mainly in animals, may be summarised as follows:

(1) Diversion of bile flow leads to a sharp rise in the rate of hepatic cholesterol synthesis.

(2) The same result follows interruption of the enterohepatic cycle by cholestyramine therapy or ileal bypass.

(3) Expansion of the bile acid pool by feeding bile acids depresses hepatic cholesterol synthesis.

(4) *In vitro,* adding bile acids to the incubation medium has been reported to inhibit the incorporation of acetate into cholesterol and mevalonate by liver preparations.

Recently, Dietschy & Wilson [149] have argued persuasively against bile salts and in favour of lymph cholesterol as the controlling factor, mainly on the following grounds:

(1) Points (1) and (2) above merely relate control to the integrity of the enterohepatic circulation, not to bile salts *per se.* Impairment of the enterohepatic cycle necessarily leads to reduced absorption of cholesterol. Similarly, point (3) above may be explained by increased absorption of cholesterol.

(2) Obstruction to bile flow results in as much enhancement of cholesterol synthesis as bile diversion, although it increases the concentration of bile salts in the blood and liver.

(3) Highly purified conjugated bile salts do *not* inhibit cholesterol synthesis by liver slices *in vitro.* The inhibitory effect of unconjugated bile acids is probably non-specific and is liable to mislead when impure conjugated bile salt preparations are used.

(4) In animals with external biliary diversion the intravenous or intraduodenal infusion of pure bile acids does not prevent the rise in hepatic cholesterol synthesis.

(5) Diversion of intestinal lymph enhances cholesterol synthesis as much as bile diversion, and the effect can be prevented by infusing chylomicrons containing a physiological amount of cholesterol.

References to the original experiments and more detailed discussion are to be found in references 149 and 692. It may also be added that the cholesterol-cholesterol feedback hypothesis agrees with the known inhibitory effect of dietary cholesterol [149].

SUMMARY OF THE FUNCTIONS OF BILE SALTS IN RELATION TO CHOLESTEROL

The very intimate relationship between bile salts and cholesterol is expressed in six main ways.

(1) As the major end product of cholesterol metabolism, bile salts provide an important excretory pathway for cholesterol. Bile salt excretion probably accounts for about 40 per cent of cholesterol turnover [149].

(2) Absorbed bile salts exert negative feedback on their own synthesis, hence on cholesterol breakdown.

(3) Bile salts promote, to some extent at least, the biliary secretion of cholesterol and are essential for maintaining cholesterol in solution in the bile.

(4) Bile salts are necessary for intestinal absorption of cholesterol: (a) they are essential for solubilising cholesterol in the lumen of the intestine; (b) they may promote mucosal esterification of absorbed cholesterol prior to incorporation into chylomicrons; (c) they are necessary for hydrolysis of any esterified cholesterol in the intestinal lumen by pancreatic cholesterol esterase.

(5) The control of hepatic cholesterol synthesis is intimately connected with the enterohepatic circulation of bile salts, probably because the latter determines the availability of bile salts for promoting cholesterol absorption.

(6) Bile salts control intestinal cholesterol synthesis.

It may be added that in some species, such as the rat [701] and the dog [2], but not in man [287, 527, 702] or the rabbit [287], an increased dietary intake of cholesterol results in a rise in bile acid synthesis. This may be regarded as a compensatory effect which prevents excessive accumulation of cholesterol in the body.

OTHER EFFECTS OF BILE SALTS ON
SMALL BOWEL FUNCTION

Calcium absorption. There is good evidence from animal experiments that bile salts enhance the absorption of calcium [386, 688], possibly because the binding of calcium ions to bile salt micelles increases the total amount of calcium ions in solution [307] or because bile salts increase the solubility of calcium in the lipid cell membrane [688]. However, sequestration of bile salts by cholestyramine administration had no obvious effect on calcium absorption [660], so the physiological significance of this phenomenon is uncertain.

Iron absorption. It has been reported that bile salts enhance the absorption of sparingly soluble iron phosphates [689].

Cleansing and antisepsis. The fact that bile salts are detergents has prompted the suggestion that they may play a role in detaching particulate material from the surface of the intestinal mucosa [307]. Since bile salts also inhibit the growth of many, especially grampositive, bacteria [619], it is tempting to speculate that the relative sterility of the small intestine is due partly to bile salts. This would agree with the rapid increase in bacterial flora in the terminal ileum, since this is the area where the intestinal bile salt concentration falls most rapidly. However, Floch *et al.* have recently shown that it is only the free bile acids which significantly inhibit the growth of anaerobes *in vitro* [190]. This is odd since it is the anaerobes which are the main deconjugators.

BILE SALTS AND THE FUNCTION OF THE COLON

The main function of the colon is to extract water and electrolytes from the faecal stream. In excess this activity leads to constipation. It is possible that bile salts act physiologically to prevent undue dehydration of the faeces [197], especially since oral administration of cholestyramine to normal subjects does tend to cause constipation. There is no doubt that bile salts have laxative properties if they enter the colon in excess. This is most clearly demonstrated by the effects of feeding pure bile salts. After several days the re-absorptive capacity of the ileum is exceeded and a mild to severe diarrhoea results [307, 656]. Pathologically, bile salt catharsis occurs in disorders of the terminal ileum and possibly in non-specific diarrhoea (see Chapters 10 and 13).

The laxative activity of bile salts has two known mechanisms. First, they influence the motility of the colon *in vivo* [207] and the contraction of colonic muscle strips *in vitro* [431]; given as an enema to dogs they cause prompt defaecation [262]. Second, they inhibit colonic reabsorption of water and electrolytes. Free bile acids, especially deoxycholic, have been shown to block absorption of water and sodium from ligated loops of rat colon in concentrations as low as 1 mM [197]. Free dihydroxy bile acids inhibit absorption of sodium, chloride, potassium and water from the perfused colon of man and the dog in 3-5 mM concentrations [427, 428]. Of less physiological but great clinical interest is the fact that conjugated bile salts in 10 mM concentrations have the same effect on the human colon [428, 429]. Conjugated deoxycholate is as inhibitory as free deoxycholate. All these changes are reversible. In man there is actual secretion of sodium, potassium and water into the colonic lumen, reflecting a greater change in exsorption than in insorption [428]. Before applying these results too closely to the physiological situation it should be remembered that normally bile acids do not enter the colon in pure aqueous solution but in the complex 'mush' of ileal effluent. The rate at which they enter the colon and their physical state, including the degree of binding to solid matter, are unknown but probably important determinants of any laxative action they may have. Vegetable fibre in the diet probably promotes the passage of bile salts into the colon [10, 256, 293, 525] and it may well be that the laxative action of plant fibre and of artificial bulk-forming agents is mediated through a mild bile salt malabsorption.

9 Bile Salt Deficiency and Bile Salt Toxicity

The two main ways in which bile salts contribute to disease processes are by being quantitatively deficient and by being toxic. Toxicity may be due either to the formation of toxic metabolites or to the presence of bile salts in areas of the body not equipped to deal with them. In practice these mechanisms tend to overlap in various complex ways. A simple unifying concept which helps in the understanding of many of these disorders is 'the importance of keeping bile salts in their place'. This concept, elaborated by the author in another place [279], is essentially as follows. Within the narrowly defined limits of the enterohepatic circulation, bile salts are useful and necessary to health. If they transgress these boundaries their detergent properties may well have harmful effects on parts of the body not adapted to their presence. Furthermore, their escape from the enterohepatic circuit may result in their deficiency within the circuit. This concept is best illustrated by ileal disorders. Here, escape of excessive quantities of bile salts into the colon results not only in toxic effects on the colon but also in bile salt deficiency in the bile because of the limited compensatory capacity of liver synthesis.

Bile Salt Deficiency

The two places where bile salts are undoubtedly necessary are in the bile itself and in the lumen of the upper small intestine. Deficiency in the bile is likely if not bound to cause cholesterol insolubility and precipitation, and is probably a major factor in the genesis of cholesterol-rich gallstones. It may also be associated with reduced flow

113

of bile. Deficiency in the upper small intestine is, of course, a necessary consequence of deficiency in the bile. It may, however, be contributed to by additional factors, namely impaired emptying of the biliary tract and bacterial wastage by deconjugation. It gives rise to malabsorption of lipids, especially fat-soluble vitamins. It is most obviously exemplified by the steatorrhoea and hypo-vitaminosis D and K of patients with obstructive jaundice.

DEFINITION OF BILE SALT DEFICIENCY

Bile salt deficiency is difficult to define. In the strict sense of total body deficiency it should be definable in terms of the size of the bile salt pool. However, a glance at Table 7.1 shows how variable this measurement is even in normal subjects on a strictly controlled diet, for example 1.87-5.49 g in the study of Hellström and Lindstedt [289]. The most recent and complete investigation of 'normal' pool sizes, that of Vlahcevic and colleagues from Richmond, Virginia [684], showed that the total bile salt pool ranges down to 1.68 g, but adding two standard deviations to their mean value of 2.37 g gives a 'normal range' of 1.37-3.17 g. On the other hand, the same group have estimated the dividing line between lithogenic and non-lithogenic bile to rest on a bile salt pool size of about 1.6-1.8 g [637].

If cholelithiasis is indeed due to bile salt deficiency then it may be said to be the first clinical indicator of such a deficiency. It is presumably a more sensitive index than lipid malabsorption since there is no evidence that patients with gallstones have steatorrhoea or even difficulty in absorbing fat-soluble vitamins.

From the functional point of view, the diagnosis of bile salt deficiency should perhaps rest on the ratio of bile salt to cholesterol in the bile and on the concentration of bile salts in the intestinal lumen during digestion. Unfortunately the normal ranges for these values are not clearly defined. In the case of the bile salt/cholesterol ratio it is questionable whether a normal range is obtainable in the Western population. The incidence of cholelithiasis is so high that many apparently normal people are in a pre-gallstone state and so probably have abnormal bile. Indeed in populations with a very high incidence of gallstones (Scandinavians and American Indians) many 'control' subjects have bile which is supersaturated with cholesterol [116, 469, 656, 680], and some of these subjects have been shown to have a reduced bile salt pool [680]. For a truly normal range it is probably necessary to examine populations where gallstones are rare or unknown. In Africans, who rarely get gallstones, the limited studies so far done show the bile salt/cholesterol ratio to be significantly higher than in Western subjects [46, 408]. Thus, in East African Masai the ratio was 25.4 ± 11.4, whereas in New Zealanders it was 17.3 ± 8.1, in Americans 13.7 ± 6.0 and in Finns 8.6 ± 2.3 [46]. It remains to be seen whether these ratios correlate with bile salt pool sizes.

It is also difficult to define the normal lower limit for the concentration of bile salts in the upper small bowel because of the extremely variable results obtained in normal subjects. Values as low as 2-2.5 mM may be observed, although the mean value is around 10 mM [191, 594] and very few are below 4 mM [191]. In patients with ileal resection, whose steatorrhoea is considered to be related to bile salt deficiency, the post-prandial jejunal bile salt concentration almost always falls below 4 mM for some if not most of the time [373, 419, 673]. Van Deest and his colleagues [673] chose a bile salt concentration of 1.7 mg/ml or approximately 3.5 mM as a useful dividing line. This figure corresponded with a micellar phase fat concentration of 0.8 mg/ml, which was exceeded by only one out of 11 samples from ileectomy patients with steatorrhoea, but by 33 out of 42 samples from control subjects.

The figure of 4 mM was chosen by Badley and colleagues [19] as the 'critical physiological concentration' on the basis of *in vitro* experiments. They incubated intestinal aspirate containing 3.5 mM bile salts with a lipid mixture (after lipase inactivation), and found that very little lipid was taken into micellar solution. On the other hand, another aspirate containing 5.5 mM bile salts dissolved almost as much lipid as one containing 11.5 mM bile salts. The difference between the critical physiological concentration and the critical micellar concentration of a similar mixture, which is about 1.5 mM, is due to the need to form a sufficiently large number of micelles to dissolve the hydrolytic products of a normal dietary lipid intake [19]. An interesting additional finding in this study was that adding excess lipid caused the amount of lipid in micellar solution to fall, suggesting that if a micelle is expanded too much it may be disrupted.

It is doubtful if bile salt deficiency ever occurs as an isolated abnormality, except possibly in cholelithiasis. As a cause of steatorrhoea it is usually associated with other abnormalities such as rapid intestinal transit in ileectomy, formation of toxic free bile acids in the stagnant loop syndrome, and possible malfunction of the gallbladder and pancreas in cirrhosis of the liver.

CAUSES OF BILE SALT DEFICIENCY

For practical purposes the causes of bile salt deficiency can be classified into two main groups:

A. *Bile salt pool reduced but no lipid malabsorption*
   Cholelithiasis [517, 679, 680], perhaps due to impaired cholesterol catabolism.
B. *Bile salt deficiency associated with lipid malabsorption*
   (1) Ileal resection or bypass.
   (2) Stagnant loop syndrome.
   (3) Vagotomy (and gastro-jejunostomy).
   (4) Biliary obstruction.
   (5) Hepatic cirrhosis.

Each of these disorders, except vagotomy, will be considered in detail in the next three chapters.

Vagotomy, especially when associated with gastro-enterostomy, has been shown to cause low concentrations of bile salts in the postprandial intestinal aspirate, together with some evidence of reduced formation of a micellar phase and of delay in fat absorption [187]. Decreased concentrations of lipase were also noted and these, together with rapid intestinal transit, may well be additional contributants to the mild steatorrhoea sometimes observed after vagotomy and drainage procedures.

Bile Salt Toxicity

TOXICITY DUE TO BILE SALTS 'IN THE WRONG PLACE'

In the following diseases there is reason to believe that bile salts may be pathogenic through their effects, detergent or otherwise, on organs not adapted to their presence: gastritis and gastric ulcer, pancreatitis, diarrhoea associated with ileal disease or resection, some cases of non-specific diarrhoea, some of the features of cholestasis (pruritus, bradycardia, target cells). These conditions will be discussed in Chapters 10-13.

TOXICITY DUE TO ABNORMAL FORMATION
OR PERSISTENCE OF TOXIC METABOLITES

There are no diseases which have been unequivocally attributed to the toxic action of bile salt metabolites but in certain conditions there is reason to suspect such a mechanism. In the stagnant loop syndrome, some of the diarrhoea and malabsorption may be due to the effect of deconjugated bile acids on small intestinal function. In chronic liver disease, cholestasis and disseminated sclerosis there is circumstantial evidence to implicate the toxicity of lithocholic acid. There are theoretical reasons to suspect a carcinogenic effect of degraded bile acids in the aetiology of carcinoma of the colon.

All these diseases will be discussed in later chapters.

Because they may be involved in a variety of disorders, the general properties and effects of free bile acids and of lithocholate will be discussed in the following sections.

THE TOXICITY OF FREE OR DECONJUGATED BILE ACIDS
(EXCLUDING LITHOCHOLIC ACID)

In recent years there has been much interest in the properties and effects of free bile acids, mainly because of the association of excessive bile salt deconjugation in the small intestine with malabsorption. Consequently most investigators have studied the effects of free bile acids on the intestinal mucosa.* Their findings may be summarised as follows:

(1) With *in vitro* preparations all three free bile acids, cholic, deoxycholic and chenodeoxycholic, are inhibitory to the main active *transport systems* in the jejunum, namely those for glucose, amino acids and sodium. However, there is a marked difference in inhibitory potency, cholate being active only at concentrations of 5 mM and above, but deoxycholate and chenodeoxycholate having marked effects at 0.2 or 0.25 mM [23, 197, 518]. The latter effect is so great as to be apparent with unpurified commercial preparations of conjugated bile salts

---

* Less clinically orientated investigators have concentrated on the haemolytic properties of free bile acids [349]. Whichever cytotoxic action is studied it is found that the toxicity of a bile acid is inversely proportional to the number of hydroxyl groups on its steroid nucleus [349].

contaminated with deoxycholate [518]. Rather ironically, at concentrations above 0.5 mM deoxycholate even inhibits the bile salt transport system in the ileum [320].

(2) Similarly, with *in vitro* preparations, all *metabolic processes* so far studied are inhibited strongly by free bile acids, especially deoxycholate. These include such fundamental activities as oxygen utilisation, ATPase activity and synthesis of protein, triglyceride and sterols [102, 135, 144, 151, 518]. Likewise, with liver preparations, unconjugated especially dihydroxy bile acids markedly depress a number of metabolic processes [137, 140, 381]. All this suggests that deoxycholate and chenodeoxy-cholate are non-specific metabolic inhibitors or cell poisons, and it is noteworthy that deoxycholate has been used in the laboratory to break up cell fractions. The greater cytotoxicity of the dihydroxy bile acids may reflect their greater surface activity [160], their lesser solubility or their tendency to adsorb to tissue solids [320]. It has been shown that within the liver cell deoxycholate has a marked tendency to bind to mito-chondria and microsomes [488]. On the other hand, the toxic effects of dihydroxy bile acids on hepatic microsomes have been reproduced by synthetic detergents, suggesting that it is the surface activity of the bile acids which is pathogenic [140], at least in the liver.

(3) The cytotoxicity of free bile acids *in vitro* can also be demonstrated under the microscope. Low-Beer and his col-leagues found there was excessive shedding of obviously injured epithelial cells from villous tips when small intestinal loops of hamsters or guinea-pigs were incubated for 60 min with 2.5 mM deoxycholate or chenodeoxycholate or with 5mM cholate [412]. Even more extensive damage with loss of whole villi was noted by Dawson & Isselbacher [135], while Donaldson [151] and Holt [320] found changes at deoxycholate concentrations of only 0.6 mM and 1.0 mM respectively.

(4) With *in vivo* studies a rather different pattern emerges. If intestinal segments are perfused with solutions containing deoxycholate or chenodeoxycholate 1.2 mM but no conjugated bile salts, it is still possible to show villous damage (usually more in the proximal than distal small intestine) [412] and also inhibition of those metabolic functions such as fatty acid

esterification which involve membrane-bound enzymes [102, 144]. However, when normal levels of conjugated bile salt are present (for example 15 mM taurocholate with 2 mM deoxycholate) the anti-metabolic effect of deoxycholate is completely abolished [101, 144]. This may be because, when deoxycholate is incorporated into micelles of conjugated bile salt, its intraluminal activity is decreased and its rate of absorption is slower [144]. After *in vivo* perfusion studies, the mucosal concentration of deoxycholate is much lower than after *in vitro* incubations [101], but this must be due partly to the fact that *in vitro* there is no circulating blood to remove absorbed materials.

It is tempting to dismiss all the above-mentioned *in vitro* demonstrations of bile salt toxicity as artefacts, with no relevance to the clinical situation. This, however, would be a premature judgement. In rats with experimental blind loops, bile salt deconjugation is associated with transport defects for water-soluble materials [23, 235], which can obviously not be attributed to deficiency of conjugated bile salts. Gracey *et al.* have shown that the impairment of sugar transport in such rats is greatest where there is most bile salt deconjugation [235]. A direct effect of the bacteria cannot be the cause since the effect is absent in bile-diverted rats [23]. Indeed, *in vivo* perfusion experiments have clearly shown 1 mM deoxycholate to inhibit transport systems for monosaccharide sugars [234]. Overall, therefore, there are good reasons for suspecting that free dihydroxy bile acids can be pathogenic *in vivo*.

(5) When a diet containing 2 per cent deoxycholate was fed to mice, there was in the first few days marked oedema and cellular exfoliation of the small intestinal villi. However, after 39 days the intestinal mucosa was virtually normal [205]. Other rats fed deoxycholate 25 mg daily had morphologically normal intestinal villi [583]. It has been stated [134] that feeding deoxycholate to rats does not produce steatorrhoea. These various observations suggest again that deoxycholate is non-toxic when there are enough conjugated bile salt micelles available to mask and dilute it. Deoxycholate feeding will after a few days lead to a marked expansion of the bile salt pool with conjugated deoxycholate.

Experience with feeding free dihydroxy bile acids to man is limited. In doses of 1200 mg/day they are said to cause anorexia [69]; other effects were not reported. Chenodeoxycholic acid 750-1000 mg/day caused only 'an occasional slight increase in stool frequency' [656]; no small bowel investigations were carried out, but the diarrhoea was probably due only to increased passage of bile salts into the colon. This bile acid has been administered daily for a full year without obvious toxicity [127]. However, as Small has pointed out, chenodeoxycholate feeding may well cause cholesterol to accumulate in the body [605].

Possible toxic effects of free bile acids on the liver (in cholestasis), the gallbladder, pancreas and stomach are considered in Chapters 11-13.

LITHOCHOLIC ACID

Lithocholic (3α-hydroxy-5β-cholanoic) acid is uniquely interesting to clinicians because of its extreme toxicity. It is also interesting in its own right as the only mono-hydroxy bile acid identified in human bile, which has quite different physicochemical properties to the other bile acids, and which has a special metabolic pathway, namely sulphation.

As the name implies, lithocholic acid is very insoluble in water. Its insolubility (and its high critical micellar temperature [314]) means that it does not function as a bile acid and it should perhaps not be named as such. Curiously, its glycine conjugate is less soluble than the free bile acid, and taurolithocholate is even less soluble again. Lithocholate is, however, quite freely soluble in solutions of other bile salts, presumably by being taken up into their micelles [606], as an insoluble amphiphile [314]. One part of lithocholate is solubilised by nine parts of polyhydroxylated bile salt [500]. The potassium salt is appreciably more soluble than the sodium salt. This may mean that at times lithocholate stays in solution within the liver cell but precipitates out in the sodium-rich bile [606].

Lithocholic acid is the second most abundant bile acid or bile acid derivative in human faeces [539], comprising up to 46 per cent of the total faecal bile acids [5]. It is derived by 7α-dehydroxylation of chenodeoxycholic acid [290, 484] and, with its 3-β isomer isolithocholic acid, it is the main faecal end product of chenodeoxycholic acid metabolism [124]. The formation of lithocholic acid by human faecal organisms has been demonstrated *in vitro* [252, 482], but much less is known of the capacity of individual bacterial species to produce lithocholate than is the case with deoxycholate. Lithocholate is absorbed very poorly from the colon [484, 290], perhaps because it is so insoluble. An additional factor may be its tendency to bind to bacteria and other solid matter [252, 482], especially since it is well absorbed from the caecum of germ-free rats [257]. In fact, small but significant quantities are absorbed in man since lithocholate is regularly present in normal bile. Indeed the size of the lithocholate pool has been estimated indirectly in 10 American male hospital patients as 0.05 ± 0.02 g (range 0.01-0.07 g) [684]. This represents just over 2 per cent of the total bile salt pool on average, but in one subject it was over 4 per cent. Litho cholic acid has also been identified in the blood of two normal subjects [93], but it is not able to be quantified in the blood by current techniques [503, 549].

In the bile lithocholate is probably carried in the mixed micelles, since after electrophoresis it and its metabolites are found in the macromolecular complex [481].

Unlike the other secondary bile salt deoxycholate, lithocholate is metabolised beyond simple conjugation with glycine and taurine. This was first suspected when, in the bile of two patients who had been given labelled lithocholate orally, more than half the radioactivity was found in metabolites which were much more polar then glyco- or taurolithocholate [481]. Palmer went on to identify these substances as the 3α-sulphates of the two conjugates and to confirm that these constituted about half the biliary metabolites of lithocholate [499]. This esterification of the 3α-hydroxyl group is of great theoretical interest because it is analogous to the sulphation of bile alcohols, the primitive equivalent of bile acids found in some lower vertebrates [275]. At a more practical level, the addition of a second negative charge to the lithocholate molecule changes its biological properties profoundly. This has been clearly shown in respect of intestinal absorption [413]. Whereas both tauro- and glycolithocholate are freely absorbed from guinea-pig jejunum, their sulphates are not absorbed to any significant extent. The sulphates are absorbed from the ileum by the active transport system, but at this point they are subject to competition with other bile salts for the limited number of transport sites [413]. The implication is that sulphation limits the mechanism for reabsorbing and so retaining lithocholate. This in turn suggests that sulphation is essentially a detoxication process. Certainly other toxic steroids are detoxicated by sulphation [499]. There is preliminary evidence in rats that sulphation does reduce the toxic effects of lithocholate on bile canaliculi [189].

The site of lithocholate sulphation has not been proved. Logically it should be the liver, but this is hard to reconcile with the finding of Carey & Williams that the biles of two patients given lithocholic acid-24-^{14}C intravenously contained almost all their radioactivity in glyco- and taurolithocholate [92]. Possibly more than one passage through the liver is required. On the other hand, other steroid sulphates can be synthesised in the intestine [499].

Minute quantities of lithocholic acid are secreted into the bile unconjugated [92]. Isolithocholate, which is made by bacteria from lithocholate, has also been detected in the bile [481], but its absorption is even more limited than that of lithocholate, possibly because it is esterified in the colon with fatty acids [481].

The livers of rats [502] and hamsters [360] hydroxylate lithocholate to some extent, producing more polar and presumably less toxic compounds. The fact that the rabbit cannot do this may explain why it is so sensitive to the toxicity of lithocholate. Man also is unable to hydroxylate lithocholate.

The toxic properties of lithocholate and its conjugates are manifold. *In vitro* they haemolyse human erythrocytes and disrupt other membranes such as those of lysosomes [500]. Injected intramuscularly into human volunteers in doses of only 6 mg, lithocholic acid caused within 12 h a fever of 103°F (39.5°C) or more, and intense malaise, fatigue, headache, anorexia and nausea [501]. In addition a marked inflammatory reaction developed at the site of injection. This reached its peak at 2-3 days, well after the fever had subsided, and sometimes took 2-4 weeks to resolve. Glycolithocholate had the same effect but taurolithocholate usually caused only the local inflammation and the systemic symptoms without the fever. Although these studies do not necessarily correlate with clinical conditions it is worth noting that the body probably contains about 50 mg of lithocholate outside the intestine [684] and only 6 mg were required to produce the effects noted above.

Currently there is much interest in the pathogenic effects of lithocholate on the liver and biliary tract. This began with the discovery of Holsti in 1956 that feeding a crude commercial bile preparation (which incidentally was available as a pharmaceutical product! [88]) to rabbits produced cirrhosis [316]. Holsti went on to identify the cirrhosis-producing agents as lithocholic and glycolithocholic acids, and their precursor chenodeoxycholic acid [317, 318]. Lithocholate injured the liver when given with the diet at a level of only 0.25 per cent. In low doses it caused predominantly bile duct changes, ductular proliferation and hyperplasia. Since these same changes can be produced in rats (provided a low-protein diet is fed, too) [95, 502], mice, hamsters, guinea-pigs [500], monkeys [327] and baboons [95], and also in birds, reptiles and amphibians [500], it is not unreasonable to suppose that lithocholate might cause liver or bile ductular damage in man (see Chapter 11).

In the rat, 1 per cent lithocholate feeding causes the formation of gallstones. These are composed mainly of the glycine conjugates of lithocholic acid and its 6β-hydroxylated derivative [95, 502], combined with the debris of sloughed-off bile ductular cells [500]. Stone formation does not occur if the diet contains sufficient sulphur-containing amino acids to permit the normal taurine conjugation of bile salts. The fact that both a low-protein diet and a high dose of lithocholate are necessary suggests that these experiments contribute little to the problem of human gallstones, which in any case are never rich in lithocholate.

There is at present much work in progress on the effects of lithocholate and its conjugates and sulphates on the finer aspects of liver function, especially bile secretion and cholesterol metabolism. When taurolithocholate is infused intravenously into rats or hamsters there is a prompt fall in bile flow. This can be prevented or reversed by simultaneous infusion of enough 'normal' micelle-forming bile salt to keep the molar ratio of other bile salt to taurolithocholate in the bile above two (in the hamster) [339]. This also hastens the biliary secretion of taurolithocholate. The explanation originally suggested for these phenomena was obstruction of small bile ducts by precipitated taurolithocholate and its prevention or relief by incorporation into micelles [339]. However, more recent work with the isolated perfused hamster liver suggests that taurolithocholate causes cholestasis by interfering with the bile salt-independent fraction of bile flow, since during cholestasis bile salt secretion was maintained but sodium output was reduced [360]. In these experiments the dose of taurolithocholate used was very small (up to 2 mg) and the liver appeared morphologically normal. In a similar study, where about 12 mg of taurolithocholate, glycolithocholate or free lithocholate were added to the perfusing solution of rat livers, electron microscopy showed significant morphological alterations involving only the bile canaliculi. These changes consisted of dilatation, loss of microvilli and reduplication of the canalicular membrane [189]. The similarity of such changes to those seen in patients with intrahepatic cholestasis, together with the presence in these patients of structures resembling liquid crystals (which could be considered as failed bile salt micelles) adjacent to the canaliculi, has led Schaffner & Popper [557] and others [215] to construct lithocholate-based hypotheses for human cholestasis (see Chapter 11).

Effects of lithocholic acid on hepatic cellular metabolism have also been noted. In a number of species, feeding lithocholate alters the plasma and liver concentrations of cholesterol and phospholipid [328, 389, 466]. In the rat, rabbit and chick the liver concentration of cholesterol is increased, and this can occur without cholestasis or any alteration in hepatic morphology [466]. Since at the same time the liver concentration of cholic acid was found to be decreased and that of chenodeoxycholic acid increased, Nair and colleagues postulated that lithocholic acid inhibits the enzyme 12α-hydroxylase [466]. This is the enzyme which directs the synthetic pathway towards cholic acid rather than chenodeoxycholic acid (see Fig. 5.1). They also suspected that lithocholate blocks the uptake of cholic acid by gut mucosa. There are therefore several ways in which lithocholic acid may alter bile salt and cholesterol metabolism.

Interest in lithocholic acid is continuing and growing. It will certainly be increased by the recent demonstration of lithocholate in the brain of a patient with multiple sclerosis [471]. For his own part, the author considers it quite probable that lithocholate is involved in the genesis of cholesterol gallstones and of ulcerative proctocolitis.

10 Diseases in which Bile Salts Play an Important Role

I. Disorders of the Terminal Ileum, and Bacterial Overgrowth in the Small Intestine

In the last few years the medical journals have contained many papers on the role of bile salts in disease. These have established that disturbed bile salt metabolism is responsible for prominent features of several diseases, most of which are quite common. These diseases are considered in this and the next two chapters. There are also at least nine common diseases in which evidence is beginning to accumulate for a pathogenic role of bile salts. These are discussed in Chapter 13. Finally there are diseases where bile salt metabolism is certainly altered but where this change is probably of no pathological significance. These are considered in Chapter 14.

Disorders of the Terminal Ileum; 'Terminal Ileopathy'

Interest in patients with ileal disorders rose sharply after it was discovered in the early nineteen-sixties that the terminal ileum has a crucial role in the enterohepatic circulation of bile salts [60, 376]. It was already known that resection of the distal small intestine causes much more diarrhoea and, if extensive, steatorrhoea than resection of the proximal small bowel [52, 346, 371], but this was interpreted as signifying that fat absorption takes place mainly in the ileum [346]. However, the intubation studies of Borgström and his colleagues established that fat is rapidly absorbed in the jejunum [59, 60]. These apparently contradictory observations were reconciled by studies of bile salt metabolism in ileectomy patients. These patients, and also those with diseased but surgically untouched terminal ileums, were found to have grossly disturbed bile salt metabolism, together with watery diarrhoea and sometimes steatorrhoea. These gastro-intestinal disturbances were blamed on dysfunction of the terminal ileum causing bile salt malabsorption. The expression 'cholerhoeic enteropathy' coined by Hofmann [306] is therefore very apt. However, other mechanisms probably contribute to diarrhoea and steatorrhoea in ileal disorders, and patients with them do display other features in common, namely a tendency to hypocholesterolaemia and to cholelithiasis [105, 285] and possibly to peptic ulceration. The author therefore prefers the expression 'terminal ileopathy' if one is required to describe this syndrome.

The abnormalities of bile salt metabolism that occur in disordɜrs of the terminal ileum may be grouped under four main headings: accelerated turnover, or malabsorption; increased amount synthesised and turned over; decreased availability (bile salt deficiency); and altered composition of the bile salt pool. In considering each abnormality I shall discuss the evidence for the defect, its presumed mechanism and its probable effects.

(1) *Accelerated turnover of bile acids. Malabsorption.* Several groups of investigators have shown that, when patients with ileal disorders are given radioactive bile salts by mouth or intravenously, they excrete the label very rapidly in their faeces [426, 622, 709], or lose it very rapidly from their duodenal aspirate [17, 270, 280, 411, 673]. All these studies except one [411] have been done using labelled cholic acid or its conjugates. However, it is improbable that significantly different results would be obtained with dihydroxy bile acids. These studies indicate that an abnormally large fraction of the bile salt pool (or, more precisely since there is no steady state, of the bile salts entering the intestine) is lost per unit of time. In other words, each time the available pool enters the intestine, far more than the normal 3 per cent or so escapes reabsorption and far less then 97 per cent returns to the liver. The precise magnitude of the defect is difficult to assess. The best estimate is probably obtained by comparing the faecal excretion rate of bile acid radioactivity with that of an unabsorbable marker such as ^{51}Cr

given simultaneously. By this means Woodbury *et al.* showed that when the entire ileum is resected or diseased there is essentially no reabsorption of cholic acid [709]. The enterohepatic circulation is totally interrupted. Similarly Low-Beer *et al.* [411] studied the effect of a single meal on the reappearance of labelled bile salt in duodenal aspirate, and found that only 2-5 per cent returned in ileectomy patients, but 70 per cent or more in normal subjects. The defect was as great with labelled glycochenodeoxycholate as with glycocholate.

With partial ileal resections extending to the ileo-caecal sphincter, there is a lesser but still severe defect of bile salt absorption. Provided 60 cm or more of ileum are resected, the loss of bile salt may be such that labelled taurocholate is virtually all lost from the bile in 24 h [278] and the cholic acid half-life (measured by faecal excretion*) is reduced from a normal mean of 6.2 days† to less than 0.5 days [426]. Even when only 40 cm of terminal ileum are diseased or resected, the coefficient of absorption of cholic acid is decreased from the normal of about 95 per cent to 64-80 per cent [709].

The *mechanism* of this malabsorption is presumably loss of active transport sites in the terminal ileum. The colon is unable to absorb a significant proportion of the bile salts pouring into it, partly no doubt due to the action of the bile salts themselves in inhibiting its absorptive functions and increasing its motility. The small bowel transit time may well be decreased, but it is unlikely that this is an important factor, since Meihoff & Kern showed that the cholic acid half-life is only slightly shortened in normal subjects suffering from mannitol-induced diarrhoea [426]. Another possible factor is bacterial proliferation in the small bowel due to loss of the protective action of the ileo-caecal sphincter. Unfortunately, systematic studies of the small bowel microflora have been performed in few patients with ileal disorders. Excessive bacterial counts and/or bile salt deconjugation have been noted occasionally [227, 373, 419], and would probably be found more often if intestinal aspirates were routinely taken for culture after meals [227]. However,

---

* The half-life cannot be determined from duodenal aspirates when the rate of loss is so great that synthesis cannot keep pace (see page 86).
† This is double the *T*½ obtained from duodenal aspirates, probably because of delay in colonic transit.

there is reason to believe that, in ileectomy patients, bacterial overgrowth actually helps to conserve bile salts. In such patients, intestinal stasis is associated with less rapid disappearance of ^{14}C radioactivity (given originally as taurocholate-24-^{14}C) [214]. There is also more dehydroxylation. This should hasten the excretion of chenodeoxycholate.

The *effects* of bile salt malabsorption are:

(a) Excessive passage of bile salts into the colon, causing watery diarrhoea. The inrushing bile salts impair absorption of water and electrolytes (possibly even causing net secretion) and may influence colonic motility directly, as discussed on page 111. The diarrhoea may be very frequent and urgent to the point of incontinence. It is usually brought on by eating or drinking, especially in the morning. There may be abdominal colic and tenesmus. The symptoms are often relieved by bile salt-sequestrating agents such as cholestyramine (see Chapter 15). In the presence of severe steatorrhoea some of the diarrhoea is probably due to the action of fatty acid soaps in the colon (cf. soap enemas) [388, 515] or to bacterially produced hydroxy fatty acids [312, 352, 357].

(b) Reduced return of bile salts to the liver. Bile acid synthesis is dis-inhibited and proceeds at a maximal rate. Overnight this may result in an accumulated 'pool' in the gall-bladder which is normal or near normal, but the loss of this 'pool' at breakfast cannot be made good by lunchtime (see below). Monkey experiments suggest that hepatic synthesis is maximal at 20 per cent interruption of the enterohepatic circulation but that at 33 per cent interruption it is inadequate to maintain bile salt secretion [154]. In complete interruption of the entero-hepatic circulation only 3.3 g (on average) of bile salts, representing maximal hepatic synthesis, can possibly enter the intestine, compared with the normal 18-24 g (6-8 entrances of a 3 g pool).

(2) *Increased amount of bile salts synthesised and turned over.* Rapid turnover cannot be equated with increased amount turned over without information on the pool size. With ileal

dysfunction, where recirculation is virtually absent, there is no miscible pool in the true sense, but merely an accumulation in the gallbladder of newly synthesised material available for the next meal. Data on the size of the overnight bile salt accumulation or 'pool' in ileectomy patients are scanty and of questionable validity (see page 90). However, in one group of four patients the 'pool' was only slightly reduced at 2.2 g [1] while in a second group of four the cholate 'pool' was 0.76 g [280], which corresponds with a total 'pool' of again about 2 g. Since isotope studies show that this 'pool' is virtually replaced within 24 h [280, 673], it follows that daily turnover cannot be less than the 'pool' size, in other words at least 2 g per day, which is four times the normal turnover rate.

More direct evidence of increased turnover has been obtained from quantitative estimation of faecal bile salts. Daily excretion rates of 1.9-4 g were present in five out of six patients with 'right ileocolectomy' reported by Fiasse et al. [186], and in all five patients with total ileal resection or disease studied by Woodbury et al. [709]. The mean bile salt excretion in Fiasse's entire group of ileum-resected patients was about 2.6 g, which is near the 3.3 g excreted by bile fistula patients, namely the maximal synthetic rate [94]. Both groups of workers found that lesser degrees of ileal damage are inconstantly associated with high excretion rates. They also found that daily faecal weight, made up mainly of water, correlates well with faecal bile acids, which suggests that the severity of diarrhoea is a rough guide to the rate of bile salt excretion and confirms the belief that the diarrhoea is 'cholegenic' in origin. In hypercholesterolaemic patients, surgical bypass of the distal third of the small intestine increases faecal bile acid excretion between four and 20 times over the pre-operative value (mean 5.8 times) [248, 449].

The *mechanism* of increased turnover has been discussed.

The *effects* of increased turnover are on the colon (as discussed opposite) and on hepatic cholesterol metabolism. In the liver the increased bile salt synthesis means of course that cholesterol catabolism is enhanced. Much of the extra cholesterol required is provided by new synthesis. It has been shown by several groups of workers [248, 449] that in hypercholesterolaemic patients subjected to ileal bypass there is a marked increase in total body synthesis of cholesterol, estimated as threefold in one study [449]. This increase has been evidenced by a more rapid decline in the specific activity of labelled plasma cholesterol and by persistently high excretion of faecal steroids. Neither phenomenon indicates where the extra cholesterol is being synthesised. There is probably a rise in intestinal cholesterol synthesis [248], and there is certainly a rise in hepatic synthesis. In monkeys, ileal bypass caused a tenfold rise in the rate of cholesterol synthesis by liver biopsies [458]. Overall, however, catabolism must be increased more than synthesis because in patients the size of the body cholesterol pool falls [449]. This helps to explain the hypocholesterolaemic effect of ileal dysfunction, which has been exploited therapeutically by Buchwald and others [76, 615]. An added factor in this effect is no doubt the malabsorption of cholesterol that follows ileal bypass [458], while with ileal resection there is also loss of the cholesterol synthetic activity of the ileum [149]. Previously normocholesterolaemic subjects with ileal dysfunction often have very low serum cholesterol levels, sometimes below 100 mg per cent [105, 153, 280, 622]. It is possible that such patients are protected from atherosclerosis, since bypass of the terminal ileum does prevent experimental atherosclerosis in monkeys [575], dogs [576] and rabbits [75]. However, most physicians wishing to lower serum cholesterol levels prefer to prescribe a 'medical ileectomy' in the form of cholestyramine [383] (see Chapter 15).

Hyperoxaluria occurs in many patients with ileal resection [155a, 315, 610a] and may be related to increased bile salt turnover. It was originally ascribed to excessive bacterial metabolism of glycine, derived from bile salt deconjugation, to glyoxylate in the colon, with hepatic conversion of glyoxylate to oxalate [315]. Certainly, feeding taurine abolishes the hyperoxaluria [155a], and it is known that this treatment reduces hepatic conjugation of bile acids with glycine [212]. However, further studies have suggested that the basic defect is inability of the liver to handle increased amounts of endogenously synthesised glyoxylate (A. F. Hofmann, personal communication).

(3) *Decreased bile salt availability (bile salt deficiency)*. When the concentration of bile salts is measured in aspirate from the upper small intestine during digestion it is usually found to be low in patients with ileal dysfunction. Four groups of workers have shown an obvious difference between ileectomy patients and normal controls in the average or maximal bile salt concentrations in the jejunum [270, 373, 419, 673]. Because of the different techniques used and the variable data obtained, it is hard to say by how much jejunal bile salt levels are reduced, but in the study of van Deest *et al.* [673], the average concentration in ileectomy patients (2.08 mg/ml, or approximately 4 mM) was exactly half that found in normal subjects. At first sight this is hard to reconcile with the rather unimpressive reduction in the size of the available pool, as estimated by isotope dilution [1, 280] (see above). However, the measurement actually made by isotope dilution is of the quantity of bile salts newly synthesised and accumulated in the gallbladder during an overnight fast. This 'pool' is largely or completely lost the first time the gallbladder contracts, and the opportunity to fill the gallbladder with a comparable amount of new bile salts does not arise till the following night. During the latter 50 per cent or more of the digestive period of any meal there will be secreted into the biliary tract only newly synthesised bile salts (assuming complete interruption of the enterohepatic circulation), so that after the initial gallbladder contraction the jejunal bile salt concentration is bound to fall sharply. Such a fall was well demonstrated by those workers who collected serial samples of intestinal aspirate after breakfast [419, 673]. After later meals the situation is worse still; the initial bile salt levels are much lower than those found at breakfast because there has been less time to accumulate newly synthesised material [673]. A possible consequence is that lipids are absorbed less well from later meals.

In ileectomy patients, intraluminal bile salt deficiency may be contributed to by two other factors: (1) Precipitation of glycine conjugates at pH levels below 4.5. There is evidence from animal experiments that ileal resection leads to increased gastric acid secretion [85, 705], and low jejunal pH values were found in some ileectomy patients by Krone *et al.* [373]. Hofmann (personal communication) has indeed found considerable precipitation of glycine conjugates in aspirates from these patients. (2) Gallbladder dysfunction may be present in the 30 per cent or so of ileectomy patients who have gallstones [285]. There is a little evidence in dogs that cholecystectomy increases the defect in fat absorption caused by ileal resection [342]. The main *mechanism* of bile salt deficiency is, however, the inability of the liver to compensate for loss of enterohepatic return, as explained on page 96.

The *effects* of bile salt deficiency in ileal dysfunction are surprisingly ill-defined. Steatorrhoea has been present in all patients reported to have low jejunal bile salt concentrations, and in nearly all of these the amount of lipid in the aqueous ('micellar') phase of intestinal content was probably reduced (when it was measured [270, 373, 673]). However, it cannot be concluded that bile salt deficiency was the sole cause or even the main cause of their steatorrhoea. Total bile diversion or obstruction causes less steatorrhoea than loss of the distal half of the small intestine. Feeding taurocholate with meals produced only a modest reduction in steatorrhoea in three of the four patients studied by Hardison & Rosenberg [270]. Woodbury & Kern [709] found no consistent relation between faecal fat and bile acid excretion. Therefore other factors must be involved. Rapid small bowel transit is probably important. Loss of both ileum and ileocaecal valve does greatly shorten intestinal transit time [426, 590], and artificially slowing it by inserting an anti-peristaltic segment reduces the malabsorption of gut-resected dogs [620]. Furthermore, D-xylose absorption is usually impaired in ileectomy patients who have steatorrhoea [186, 280], and this is most likely due to shortened contact time between xylose and small gut mucosa [192]. Other possible factors are bacterial overgrowth in the small intestine, and impaired pancreatic lipolysis due either to lipase-inactivation at acid pH or reduced bile salt stimulation of pancreatic enzyme release. Against the last two possibilities is the finding of absent triglyceride in the stool of ileectomy patients [270].

Malabsorption of fat-soluble vitamins is to be expected since these vitamins are completely dependent on bile salts for their absorption. However, the writer knows of no studies on vitamin absorption after ileal resection. Vitamin D deficiency in the form of osteomalacia is distinctly rare after intestinal resection [53, 186, 704]. Hypocalcaemia and malabsorption of calcium are commoner [186] but may just reflect the severity of the steatorrhoea.

Cholelithiasis in ileectomy patients may be due to bile salt deficiency. In the only two patients so far reported, the bile was saturated with cholesterol [105]. Experimentally, interrupting the enterohepatic circulation reduces the bile salt/cholesterol ratio [155, 662], but with chronic interruption in monkeys there is a compensatory increase in phospholipid secretion [155].

(4) *Altered bile salt patterns in the bile.* Patients with ileal dysfunction characteristically have an elevated ratio of glycine-conjugated to taurine-conjugated bile salts, or G/T ratio [280, 419]. Ratios between 10 and 20 are usual and they may approach 30 [1, 212, 285, 419], compared with a normal upper limit of 5 or 6 [212, 596]. There seems to be no correlation between the length of ileum diseased or resected and the height of the G/T ratio, at any rate when more than 60 cm of ileum is removed [213]. The fact that the ratio is also high in un-operated cases of ileal Crohn's disease [74, 212, 285] raises the possibility of using it as a screening test for ileal disease. Indeed two patients have been reported in whom a high G/T ratio was the first detectable sign of ileal Crohn's disease [74]. However, the specificity of this sign has yet to be established. It can certainly be present with bacterial overgrowth in the small intestine [645] and in tropical sprue [347], and it may be a feature of other diarrhoeal illnesses.

The *mechanism* of the altered bile salt conjugation has occasioned some disagreement. Some authors have assumed that it represents selective retention of glycine conjugates due to their absorption by passive diffusion in the jejunum [1, 419]. The only experimental basis for this belief is that in jejunal perfusion studies glycine conjugates are taken up to a significant extent whereas taurine conjugates are not [298]. However, the relevance of this finding to the clinical situation has not been demonstrated. On the other hand, Garbutt et al. [212] have clearly shown that the high G/T ratio arises within the liver. Intravenous injection of ^{14}C-labelled free deoxycholate was followed by the appearance in the duodenum of radioactive glycodeoxycholate and taurodeoxycholate in the same proportions as previously aspirated glycocholate and taurocholate. By the first theory of GDC-^{14}C/TDC-^{14}C ratio should be lower than the GC/TC ratio if part of the GC was recirculated. Furthermore, when the ratio of GDC-^{14}C to TDC-^{14}C was measured on two or three consecutive days it did not show the tendency to rise that would be expected if glycodeoxycholate is reabsorbed more efficiently than taurodeoxycholate.

It remains to be explained why the liver conjugates so much with glycine, so little with taurine. It cannot be loss of the enzymes for taurine-conjugation, since feeding taurine reduces the G/T ratio as strikingly as it does in normal subjects [212, 595]. The clue probably lies in the fact that a similar elevation of the G/T ratio occurs in two other situations where the enterohepatic circulation is interrupted and there is a great rise in bile salt synthesis, namely with bile diversion [172] and during cholestyramine therapy [282, 354]. In all three situations the raised G/T ratio can be explained as due to relative unavailability of taurine and its precursor cysteine, in the face of a much increased demand for bile acid conjugation. Taurine is much less plentiful in the body than glycine, the major physiological role of taurine being bile salt conjugation [337], whereas glycine is metabolically ubiquitous.

No important *effects* of a raised G/T ratio have been reported. Glycine conjugates are more easily precipitated than taurine conjugates by acid or calcium, but since glycine conjugates predominate even in normal subjects this is unlikely to be very important.

Alterations in the relative proportions of cholate, chenodeoxycholate and deoxycholate have been reported in ileectomy patients. Abaurre *et al.* found the cholate pool to be reduced by about half but the chenodeoxycholate pool to be unchanged [1]. Similarly McLeod & Wiggins [419] found cholate to be reduced relative to chenodeoxycholate. However, whereas Abaurre *et al.* showed the deoxycholate pool to be significantly increased, McLeod & Wiggins found deoxycholate to be reduced in one and absent in three of five patients. This discrepancy may be due to the fact that the latter but not the former patients had undergone resection of the right colon, which could shorten the colonic transit time so much that little deoxycholate is formed or absorbed.

DETECTION OF ILEAL DYSFUNCTION IN CLINICAL PRACTICE

In the clinical investigation of ileal function there are no generally available tests apart from measurements of vitamin B_{12} absorption. There are occasions when it would be helpful to be able to detect the effects of terminal ileopathy on bile salt metabolism. This can be done in several ways.

(1) The most direct and reliable test is measurement of *faecal radioactivity* after administration of labelled bile salt orally or intravenously. This has been shown to distinguish clearly between patients with ileal resection and controls [203, 426, 622] and a normal upper limit has been suggested of 20 per cent of the administered dose excreted in 24 h [203]. Some patients with unoperated ileal disease have given a positive test [203, 426] and presumably they had diarrhoea since there is a positive correlation between faecal mass and faecal bile acids [186, 709]. This test, like all quantitative stool collections, suffers disadvantages which are increased in the presence of diarrhoea. Also it requires special counting equipment. However, if this test is negative, terminal ileopathy can be excluded.

(2) An equally direct test is measurement of *bile radioactivity* after administration of labelled bile salt [280, 673]. This has the considerable disadvantage of requiring at least two duodenal intubations, which is unfortunate since it can give extra information about the metabolism of bile salts and the size of the bile salt pool [212, 214, 280].

(3) *Measurement of the ratio of glycine-conjugated to taurine-conjugated bile salts* in the bile has been advocated as a screening test for terminal ileopathy [74]. Certainly a raised G/T ratio is almost invariably present in terminal ileal disorders but its specificity has not been established. Furthermore a duodenal intubation and chromatographic separation are required.

(4) By far the simplest, quickest and most convenient test so far suggested is a *breath test*. This depends on the measurement of $^{14}CO_2$ in the expired breath after ingestion of glycine-1-^{14}C

labelled glycocholate [315]. This is, strictly speaking, a test for increased bacterial deconjugation of bile salts because positive results, that is increased $^{14}CO_2$ in the breath in the first 5 or 6 h, are given by patients with bacterial contamination of the small bowel as well as those with ileal disorders [203, 581]. Apart from a liquid scintillation counter the apparatus required is simple, cheap and versatile [546]. Fromm & Hofmann [203] have found no false positives but occasional false negatives, perhaps because of rapid colon transit or unusual bacteria which do not split glycine to CO_2. The test should be regarded as a semi-quantitative screening test and positive results need to be interpreted in the light of other data such as faecal weight, response to cholestyramine therapy and, if available, faecal ^{14}C [203].

(5) Lessening of diarrhoea (preferably monitored by stool weights) during oral *administration of cholestyramine* 4 g three or four times daily is a useful test for bile salt malabsorption [312, 515]. Patients with severe steatorrhoea do not respond well but in them the ileal disorder will probably be clinically obvious. Some patients with 'non-specific diarrhoea' also respond [541, 558] but these should give a negative breath test [203]. However, more studies are needed in these diagnostically difficult cases.

(6) High *serum levels of free bile acids* seem, on the limited data so far available [394], to be characteristic of patients with ileal resection and the stagnant loop syndrome. This could be a useful screening test in centres able to measure serum bile acids.

TREATMENT OF PATIENTS WITH ILEAL RESECTION

Diarrhoea is often reduced and sometimes abolished by *cholestyramine* therapy. Urgency, tenesmus and colic also respond [541]. The orange-flavoured preparation Questran (Bristol Laboratories) is quite pleasant to take, the usual dose being one sachet (equivalent to 4 g anhydrous cholestyramine) three or four times daily with or before meals, but a lower dose is sometimes adequate. Since therapy is likely to be life-long, care must be taken to avoid deficiency of fat-soluble vitamins (already the author has seen one patient develop osteomalacia [284]), and it is essential to give oral water-soluble or parenteral supplements of vitamins D and K, and possibly A and E, and to check plasma calcium and alkaline phosphatase regularly. A mild increase in faecal fat is likely to occur but is of no consequence. When pre-existing steatorrhoea is marked, as is likely with ileal resection or bypass of more than 100 cm, there may be a poor response to cholestyramine [312, 515], but in this case there is a good effect with dietary restriction of long chain triglycerides [515]. For nutritional reasons it may be desirable to give supplements of *medium chain triglycerides,* which are well absorbed in the absence of bile salts and therefore in the presence of cholestyramine [713].

Lignin, a natural bile salt-binding substance present in vegetable fibre (see Chapter 15), has been suggested as an alternative to cholestyramine [166]. It is certainly more palatable, but in the author's experience it is seldom as effective as cholestyramine. Its mode of action is unknown but is definitely different from that of cholestyramine [282]. Calcium carbonate is stated to relieve diarrhoea in patients with intestinal resection [388]. This may be due to precipitation of calcium salts of bile acids [312].

Administering bile salts by mouth does reduce the steatorrhoea of ileal resection but since it also exacerbates the diarrhoea [270] it has no place in therapy. The synthetic detergent Tween 80 reduces cholestyramine-induced steatorrhoea [161] and has been tried in a patient with terminal ileopathy [585], but its use must be regarded as experimental.

Bacterial Overgrowth in the Small Intestine
(The Stagnant or Blind Loop Syndrome)

After ileal disorders, the clinical disorder with bile salt involvement which has attracted the greatest interest in recent years is small bowel bacterial overgrowth, as testified to by a spate of excellent review articles [152, 233, 537, 642, 644].

The stagnant loop syndrome, or more descriptively the contaminated small bowel syndrome [233], is by definition a clinical condition characterised by malabsorption, especially of fat and vitamin B_{12}, and associated with excessive numbers of chiefly anaerobic bacteria in the small intestine. It is a heterogeneous disorder and has numerous causes, the chief ones being gastro-jejunostomy (especially with Polya gastrectomy and a large afferent loop), duodenal and jejunal diverticulosis, stricture of the small bowel as in Crohn's disease, fistula between stomach or upper small bowel and colon, surgical blind loops, scleroderma, diabetic steatorrhoea and intestinal pseudo-obstruction. All these conditions have in common one or both of two features—stasis of small bowel contents, and 'recirculation' of lower intestinal contents, which interfere with the peristaltic emptying-cleansing mechanism of the small bowel [152]. The resultant bacterial flora is very complex but tends to resemble the faecal flora [152]. The actual number of bacteria present is enormously variable, being not less than 10^4 but on occasions as high as 10^9/ml [644]. Experimental bacterial overgrowth has been produced in dogs and rats by creating blind pouches of intestine and has contributed much to our understanding of the human disorder [151, 358].

In spite of 11 years of investigation since it was first suggested by Dawson & Isselbacher that deconjugation of bile acids explains the steatorrhoea of the stagnant loop syndrome [135], the exact role of bile salts in this disorder remains disputed. It is generally agreed that, whenever there is significant malabsorption, free bile acids can be detected easily in small bowel contents, as first demonstrated in 1966 by Tabaqchali & Booth [643] and soon confirmed in man [538, 645] and dogs [358]. It is also agreed that, when careful bacteriological techniques are used, the main bacteria found are anaerobes, especially bacteroides, capable of deconjugating bile salts [159, 297]. When intestinal contents are aspirated at different levels there is usually [227] but not always [264] a correlation between the presence of bacteroides and of free bile acids. The correlation between bacterial counts and faecal fats is less good [159] but, when antibiotics are given, both the free bile acids and the bacteroides tend to disappear as the faecal fat returns to normal [227]. Antibiotics inactive against bacteroides, such as neomycin, are often ineffective clinically, whereas Lincomycin, which is particularly active against anaerobes, is effective clinically [152]. The evidence linking bacteroides and bile salt deconjugation is circumstantial (though probably as good as can be obtained), and it remains possible that bacteroides is only a marker of the stagnant conditions necessary for bile salt deconjugation [644]. Deconjugation itself is, however, the *sine qua non* of steatorrhoea in the stagnant loop syndrome.

The main source of disagreement is the question of whether

steatorrhoea is caused by the toxic action of free bile acids, especially deoxycholic, or by a reduction in the concentration of conjugated bile acids (the free acids being of little use for solubilising fat, because at the relatively acid jejunal pH they tend to precipitate or become unionised, and so fail to function as detergents). The undoubted fact that feeding taurocholate reduces the steatorrhoea [358, 645] does not solve the problem since the toxicity of free bile acids can be masked by a high concentration of conjugates [101, 144] (see page 119). The case for detergent deficiency rests largely on the finding by Tabaqchali *et al.* of low concentrations (below 5 mM) of conjugated bile salts in the upper jejunal aspirate of fasting patients [645]. The more relevant post-prandial measurements have not been reported, but the results have been linked with the data of Kim *et al.* [358], who showed that when dogs with experimental blind loops were fed a liquid fat-rich meal there was not only a lot of deconjugation but also a gross reduction of aqueous phase lipid. The argument against free bile acid toxicity is the alleged absence of morphological changes in mucosal biopsies of stagnant loop patients [152], together with the failure of deoxycholate feeding or infusion to cause permanent mucosal injury or steatorrhoea in rats [205, 644].

In favour of free bile acid toxicity (see page 117) is the fact that the steatorrhoea of bacterial overgrowth is often worse than that produced by simple bile salt deficiency as in obstructive jaundice. Secondly, contrary to previous reports, it has recently been shown that if multiple jejunal biopsies are taken there are definite if patchy abnormalities on light microscopy [7, 505], while electron microscopy shows extensive absorptive cell damage and morphologically abnormal absorption even in villi which were normal by light microscopy [7]. Similarly, rats with experimental blind loops have been shown to have patchy ultrastructural changes like those produced by deoxycholate [233]. Thirdly, no significance attaches to deoxycholate feeding [205] or infusion experiments [101, 102] unless the conjugated bile salt concentration is reduced to levels seen in patients with bacterial overgrowth. It is the author's opinion that this controversy is far from resolved.

The possible role of free bile acids in malabsorption of non-lipid substances including water and electrolytes has not been extensively investigated [233]. Baraona *et al.* showed that the jejunum of rats with experimental blind loops had an impaired transporting ability for glucose and tyrosine, unless the bile duct had been previously ligated

[23]. Gracey *et al.* have recently found that in such rats impairment of sugar transport is greatest in areas with most bile salt deconjugation [235]. They have also shown that 1 mM deoxycholate inhibits sugar transport *in vivo* [234]. These findings may have nutritional significance. Since deoxycholate inhibits the bile salt transport system itself [320], one may also speculate on the possibility of a secondary terminal ileopathy and hence bile salt catharsis, contributing to the diarrhoea of the stagnant loop syndrome. The finding by Kim *et al.* [358] of monohydroxy bile acids in blind loop dogs is provocative in view of the extreme toxicity of these substances (see page 122).

As for the fate of the free bile acids themselves remarkably little is known. Theoretically, since free bile acids are largely unionised at jejunal pH, they should be well absorbed by passive non-ionic diffusion—provided they are not precipitated or bound by bacteria. Recently Fromm & Hofmann reported normal faecal excretion of radioactivity after oral administration of ring-labelled taurocholate to five patients with bacterial overgrowth [203]. This indicates that in these patients, who did not have diarrhoea (Hofmann, personal communication), there was no significant bile salt malabsorption and is the first published evidence that the enterohepatic circulation may be intact in the stagnant loop syndrome. If this is the case it is probable that there is a jejuno-hepatic circulation rather than an ileo-hepatic circulation, the short-circuit being due to passive jejunal absorption of deconjugated bile acids.

The breath test using glycine-1-^{14}C-glycocholate (see page 135) appears to be a reliable screening test for abnormal bacterial attack on bile acids [203, 545, 581]. It seems likely that it will come into general use, in which case it will be the first bile salt test to do so. If this test is combined with measurement of faecal bile salt radioactivity it is possible to distinguish the stagnant loop syndrome from terminal ileopathy [203].

High serum levels of free bile acids were found by Lewis *et al.* in all of five patients with bacterial overgrowth [394]. This does not seem to cause pruritus or to indicate liver damage. The suggested cause is the tighter binding to plasma albumin of free over conjugated bile acids [78] in the presence of excessive absorption of free bile acids. Other possible factors include delayed hepatic transport due to shortage of side chains for conjugation (see page 61) and blocking of hepatic transport sites by slowly transported or even toxic dehydroxylated bile acids.

ENTEROLITHS

Patients with the stagnant loop syndrome occasionally form stones within the involved part of the small bowel. These stones consist mainly of free bile acids, especially deoxycholic, with fatty acids as a minor component [275]. They presumably arise through the precipitation of bacterially deconjugated bile acids, which are insoluble below pH 6.5 [156].

11 Diseases in which Bile Salts Play an Important Role

II. Cholestasis and Cirrhosis

Cholestasis (Biliary Obstruction)

The colour changes in the patient and his excreta are, of course, of diagnostic value in cholestasis. Apart from these, the main effects of cholestasis can be attributed to the failure of bile salts to enter the intestine. With intrahepatic cholestasis, the disease itself may be produced through disturbed bile salt metabolism and physiology.

EFFECTS OF CHOLESTASIS (INTRA- OR EXTRA-HEPATIC)

The moderate steatorrhoea which is invariably present is due to detergent deficiency in the small intestine. It is proportional to the depth of jaundice, and therefore presumably to the severity of cholestasis [580], though very few data are available on duodenal bile salt levels to substantiate this belief [419, 520]. Lipolysis is apparently unimpaired, but fatty acids and monoglycerides are not taken up into aqueous solution and so enter the mucosa more slowly than normal. Within the mucosa they are esterified or at least incorporated into chylomicrons more slowly than normal and the greater part of absorbed fat is carried away in the portal blood (see Chapter 8). A more serious problem is malabsorption of fat-soluble vitamins, exemplified by the common clinical problem of prolonged prothrombin time and less often a frank bleeding tendency due to vitamin K deficiency. Osteomalacia is a well-recognised complication of prolonged cholestasis and is usually attributed to malabsorption of vitamin D as well as to precipitation of calcium as fatty acid soaps [580]. Vitamin A plasma levels are low but night blindness is rare. Vitamin E deficiency may also occur but its effects are uncertain.

The assumption that malabsorption due to bile salt deficiency is the cause of osteomalacia and vitamin K deficiency has perhaps been accepted too readily. It is true that in the absence of bile negligible quantities of fat-soluble vitamins are absorbed [195]. It is also true that these conditions are treated successfully by parenteral administration of vitamins D and K. However, there are no established dietary requirements for these vitamins in adults. Vitamin D is synthesised by the skin in adequate amounts when there is normal exposure to daylight [133]. Perhaps in prolonged cholestasis the cause of vitamin D deficiency is not malabsorption but simply the fact that the patient is less likely to go out of doors. Additionally the characteristic melanin pigmentation may reduce the stimulant effect of ultraviolet light. Nutritional deficiency of vitamin K has never been recorded [133], the accepted reason being that it is synthesised by intestinal bacteria and absorbed by the host. Presumably this synthesis and absorption take place mainly in the colon. It is improbable that the detergent action of bile salts is involved in the absorption of this non-dietary vitamin K. In the lower intestine there can hardly be sufficient unabsorbed but hydrolysed fat to provide for the micellar solubilisation of a fat-soluble vitamin.

In cholestasis, failure of bile salts to enter the intestine results in their accumulation in the blood. There are few centres in which serum bile acids are measured (only two to the author's knowledge in England) but considerable information has been obtained. The fasting total bile acid level, in the recent series of Neale *et al.* [472] varied from 15.4 to 285 μM in extrahepatic obstruction and from 13.3 to 157 μM in intrahepatic cholestasis, compared with a normal range of 3.1 $\pm$ 0.7 μM. The vast majority of the serum bile acids were conjugated and the G/T ratio tended to be around 1 compared with the normal 4.2. The ratio of tri-hydroxy to di-hydroxy bile salts or T/D ratio (which because of the virtual absence of deoxycholate can be taken as synonymous with the cholate/chenodeoxycholate ratio [88]) was generally normal and was higher than the values found in cirrhosis. The last observation was also made earlier by Rudman & Kendall [543], Carey [86, 88], Rautureau *et al.* [528] and Makino *et al.* [421], but it is too inconstant to be of diagnostic value [88, 472]. If cholestasis is prolonged, the T/D ratio tends to fall, possibly because of liver damage. For a detailed account of serum bile acids in hepatobiliary disorders the reader is referred to the extensive review by Carey [88].

The urine of jaundiced patients contains measurable amounts of bile salts [240, 543], and these are probably the cause of the well-known frothiness of this urine and the tendency of flowers of sulphur to sink in it (Hay's test).

Pruritus is the most troublesome symptom in cholestasis. It is almost certainly due to retained bile acids deposited in the skin. The correlation between serum bile acid concentration and pruritus is imperfect, but four lines of evidence support a relationship between bile acids and pruritus [570]. (1) External biliary drainage relieves pruritus in patients with biliary obstruction; (2) the oral administration of ox bile or bile salts increases pruritus in patients with liver disease and causes it to return in those with biliary fistulas; (3) serum bile acids are elevated in patients with pruritic hepatobiliary disease and are on average higher in those who itch than those who do not; they are also high in pregnancy pruritus [600]; (4) cholestyramine relieves pruritus and lowers serum bile acids in most patients with incomplete biliary obstruction. However, 'since skin itches and not blood' [88] the best evidence is that provided by Schoenfield et al. [567, 570], who demonstrated high concentrations of bile acids on the skin of itching patients and in particular a fall of skin bile acids to normal on the same day as pruritus was relieved [567]. There were relatively more free bile acids and more deoxycholic acid on the skin than in the serum, but it cannot yet be said that any particular bile acid is the culprit.

Target cells in the circulating blood are a characteristic finding in obstructive jaundice. Cooper & Jandl [109] have suggested that they are due to the effect of high serum bile salts on the cholesterol in the red cell.

The hypercholesterolaemia (and hence xanthomas) which develops in biliary obstruction has not been fully explained. It is certainly associated with increased cholesterol synthesis by the liver in spite of the high bile acid concentration, and this is one of the facts which led Dietschy & Wilson to the hypothesis that hepatic cholesterol synthesis is controlled by cholesterol rather than bile acids coming from the intestine [149].

Bradycardia in obstructive jaundice has long been attributed to bile salts [613] but this problem does not seem to have been investigated by modern methods.

THE PATHOGENESIS OF CHOLESTASIS AND CONSEQUENT LIVER DAMAGE: A POSSIBLE ROLE FOR BILE SALTS

The fact that lithocholate and its conjugates are so potent at producing cholestasis in experimental animals, as discussed in Chapter 9, has provoked much speculation as to the possible role of lithocholate in human cholestasis. As a primary agent there is little to incriminate it; in patients with inflammatory bowel disease and liver dysfunction there is no excess of lithocholate in the blood [88, 472]. However, Schaffner & Popper [557] have made out a plausible case for a secondary role of lithocholate, perpetuating cholestasis and contributing to secondary liver damage. They assume that the primary agent, be it virus, drug or even extrahepatic obstruction, selectively damages the hepatocyte so that the smooth endoplasmic reticulum (SER) is affected more than the mitochondria. The SER responds by becoming hypertrophic (as actually occurs in cholestasis) and yet hypoactive in terms of its enzymatic activity, which includes ring hydroxylation of cholesterol. If the latter is inhibited, it is possible that bile acid synthesis will take place largely by the minor side-chain-oxidised-first pathway, which leads to chenodeoxycholate and which may include lithocholate as an intermediate (see Chapter 5). Alternatively, if there is selective inhibition of 12α-hydroxylation, this will direct bile acid synthesis towards chenodeoxycholate rather than cholate (see page 53) and if excess chenodeoxycholate is produced there is more chance of lithocholate being formed in and absorbed from the colon (assuming, of course, that cholestasis is incomplete). In either event, lithocholate in the liver cell could initiate a vicious circle—lithocholate damaging the SER, and the SER responding by producing more lithocholate (or its precursor). The result of all this is diminished synthesis of bile salts and accumulation of lithocholate which, in the absence of abundant bile salt micelles, tends to separate out as a liquid crystalline phase. Schaffner & Popper see cholestasis as essentially a failure of micelle formation and claim to have seen in the hepatocytes and canaliculi of cholestatic livers irregular lamellated structures which could be liquid crystals. The retained lithocholate causes inflammation and fibrosis of small bile ducts which aggravates and prolongs the cholestasis.

There is evidence to support this theory from rat experiments. Nair *et al.* [466] found that feeding lithocholate caused a rise in liver cholesterol levels and a marked fall in the cholate/chenodeoxycholate ratio in liver and bile, which suggests inhibition of 12α-hydroxylation. The work of Dean & Whitehouse [137] showed that microsomal (SER) hydroxylation of cholesterol is inhibited *in vitro* by glycodeoxycholate, and in view of other work there is little doubt that inhibition would have been greater with free bile acids and with the least hydroxylated bile acids [381].

Recently an unsaturated monohydroxy bile acid has been identified in the blood and bile of patients with intrahepatic cholestasis (G. M. Murphy, 1972, personal communication), and similar 'abnormal' bile acids have been reported in the urine of infants with biliary atresia [421a]. It remains to be seen whether this metabolic defect is part of the cause or simply an effect of cholestasis.

Currently emphasis is shifting towards the toxicity of retained di-hydroxy bile acids. Denk *et al.* have shown that dihydroxy bile acids are especially potent, probably because of their greater detergency, at damaging a major component of microsomes, cytochrome P-450 [140]. It is therefore of particular interest that bile duct ligation in rats is followed by a rise in the liver concentration of di-hydroxy bile acids to 0.3-0.6 mM, which is well within the range found to damage cytochrome P-450 *in vitro* [241]. Doubtless studies will soon be published of bile acid concentration in liver biopsies from patients with cholestasis.

The fact that phenobarbitone therapy improves patients with intrahepatic cholestasis [3, 624], relieving their pruritus and reducing their serum bile acids, is of theoretical as well as practical interest since phenobarbitone is known to induce microsomal hydroxylating enzymes. Its action in promoting plasma clearance and biliary secretion of bile salts may be explained in one of two ways, depending on whether one believes that its action is on bile salt synthesis [530] or on the bile salt-independent fraction of bile secretion [43]. Firstly, it may act by restoring normal cholesterol catabolism with full hydroxylation of steroid rings, which allows the formation of adequate bile salts to form micelles, and therefore to renewal of bile secretion which washes out the accumulated toxic bile acids. Alternatively its action may be due entirely to a washout effect through increased secretion of the bile salt-independent fraction of bile secretion.

Cirrhosis of the Liver

In the last few years many abnormalities of bile salt metabolism have been uncovered in patients with cirrhosis. The significance of these abnormalities is not always clear, nor is it possible to present a comprehensive scheme for bile salt pathophysiology in cirrhosis which explains all the observed phenomena. In this situation it is best perhaps to list briefly the abnormalities which have been reported before suggesting their causes.

ABNORMALITIES OF BILE SALTS OR THEIR METABOLISM OBSERVED IN CIRRHOSIS

(1) After intravenous injection of labelled cholic acid [51, 351, 700] or chenodeoxycholic acid [700] there is delayed clearance of radioactivity from the blood, the plasma $T\frac{1}{2}$ being 2-3 times longer than the normal of about 12 min. Moreover the radioactivity tends to reappear in the blood, especially at meal times or when cholecystokinin is injected to make the gallbladder contract, presumably because of shunting of portal blood into the systemic circulation [351].

(2) Blum & Spritz [51] used the persistence of plasma radioactivity to measure the cholic acid pool size and found it to be increased to three times normal. This, it should be noted, is the total body pool, not the enterohepatically circulating pool.

(3) Total serum bile acids are consistently raised [86, 421, 472, 494, 528, 543], though not as much as in obstructive jaundice. An increased proportion of unconjugated bile acids has been reported by some workers [421, 543], but not by others [472]. There is a higher proportion of taurine conjugates [472, 700], and of di-hydroxy bile acids [86, 421, 472, 494, 528, 543] than is found in obstructive jaundice. The relatively low tri-hydroxy/di-hydroxy ratio is consistent to the extent that 81 per cent of patients with cirrhosis have a ratio less than 1, whereas 82 per cent of patients with cholestasis have a ratio greater than 1

[88]. The ratio appears to have some prognostic value since ratios of less than 1 are almost invariable when there is much liver cell failure, but often rise when for example an alcoholic stops drinking [88]. In coma or pre-coma cholate may be undetectable [88]. It should be added that when the serum bile acid level is raised for any reason the di-hydroxy fraction is virtually all chenodeoxycholate [88].

(4) Analysis of the bile acids in bile has consistently shown a marked reduction in deoxycholate, often to unmeasurable levels [596, 669, 682]. Vlahcevic *et al.* [683] found the mean deoxycholate pool to be only 40 mg compared with 310 mg in controls. The G/T ratio tends to be low [669], but there is considerable overlap with normal [596]. This phenomenon was first noted with liver biopsies *in vitro* [170].

(5) The size of the enterohepatically circulating bile salt pool has been shown by kinetic studies to be half the normal size [683]. Vlahcevic *et al.* found the cholate pool to be reduced more than the chenodeoxycholate one but the cholate pool was still marginally the larger of the two [683]. Similarly in another study the cholate pool exceeded the chenodeoxycholate pool [700]. This is in contrast to the systemic blood pattern where chenodeoxycholate tends to predominate. The half-life of biliary bile acids is sometimes prolonged and the daily synthesis rate is low. This applies to both primary bile acids, and the total daily synthesis rate is less than half normal [683].

(6) Duodenal bile salt concentrations during the digestion of a test meal were found by Badley *et al.* [20] to be low in non-alcoholic cirrhotic patients who had steatorrhoea, but normal in those without steatorrhoea. Low levels were associated with decreased concentrations of lipid in the aqueous phase of intestinal content. These authors suggested duodenal bile salt deficiency as a major factor in the steatorrhoea of cirrhosis. However, in alcoholic cirrhosis, there is less evidence to implicate bile salt deficiency [700] and more to implicate pancreatic dysfunction [409, 425].

(7) An abnormal pattern of bile salt secretion into the duodenum was noted by Turnberg & Grahame [669], namely high resting bile flow and bile salt secretion rates, but a much reduced response to cholecystokinin. These findings suggested gall-

bladder dysfunction, and similar results were obtained in cholecystectomy patients (and by other workers in cholecystectomised dogs [463]). High bile flow rates are also found in cirrhotics with T-tube drainage [387].

SIGNIFICANCE OF BILE SALT CHANGES IN CIRRHOSIS

The fact that there is a small enterohepatic pool in the presence of a large excess of circulating bile salts (which may even constitute a larger than normal pool size [51]) suggests that there is a serious defect in transfer of bile salts from blood into bile. This defect, which may affect chenodeoxycholate more than cholate, is probably due to difficulty of secretion by regeneration nodules lacking a proper bile drainage system. Uptake of injected isotope from systemic blood is slow but the fact that the isotope has been diluted into a large systemic pool may mean that the absolute rate of bile salt clearance is normal or even increased. Similarly, reduced conjugating activity should not necessarily be inferred from slow conjugation of injected labelled cholic acid [51] and excess of free bile acids in the plasma [421]. However, there certainly seems to be a tendency to return to the foetal (? primitive) pattern of dominant taurine conjugation [173, 514].

There has been much speculation about the significance of the relative excess of chenodeoxycholate in the blood, in relation to the ability of the bacterial metabolite of chenodeoxycholate, lithocholate, to induce cirrhosis in experimental animals (see Chapter 9). Carey suggested that lithocholate might be produced in damaging excess in human cirrhosis [95]. However, we now know that the amount of chenodeoxycholate actually entering the intestine, that is the enterohepatic pool, is less than normal [683] and the amount of lithocholate in the enterohepatic pool is normal or less than normal [682, 683]. This makes Carey's theory unlikely and the onus is now on its proponents to demonstrate raised levels of lithocholate in cirrhotic livers.

The reduction of deoxycholate must imply decreased exposure of bile salts to bacteria. This is strange if, as suggested, the gallbladder's reservoir function is impaired, because patients with cholecystectomy tend to have a relative excess of deoxycholate [517]. Reduced deoxycholate might be due, at least in part, to the fact that the cirrhotic secretes only a fraction of his cholate pool into the intestine where it faces any risk of dehydroxylation. A sterile small intestine cannot be invoked since there is if anything an increase in the bacterial flora [224].

The high basal flow rate of bile and increased T-tube drainage may be due to failure of inactivation by the liver of choleretic hormones such as secretin. This problem will no doubt soon yield to radio-immunoassay.

12 Diseases in which Bile Salts Play an Important Role

III. Cholelithiasis and Cholecystitis

PATHOGENESIS OF GALLSTONES

In advanced societies the great majority of gallstones have cholesterol as their main component [633] and arise within the gallbladder. The problem of gallstone formation is therefore to a large extent the problem of why solid cholesterol accumulates in the gallbladder, and it is on this aspect that the present chapter, like most current research, will concentrate. The presence in bile of cholesterol in a solid state, or more precisely in a crystalline phase, shows that at some time in the past the capacity of the bile to dissolve cholesterol was exceeded. This capacity resides within the bile salt and lecithin fractions of the bile, which combine to disperse the otherwise insoluble cholesterol in mixed micelles, as described in Chapter 3 and depicted in Fig. 3.12. A super-saturated or *lithogenic bile* is one containing too much cholesterol relative to its content of bile salt and lecithin. Production of such bile is presumably the first stage in gallstone formation, the second being nucleation and precipitation of cholesterol crystals and the third being the enlargement of crystals by growth or agglomeration (at which stage other factors such as mucus may be concerned) [64, 603].

Cholesterol excess cannot be defined in terms of an absolute concentration of cholesterol but only in terms of the relative proportions of cholesterol, bile salts and lecithin. It cannot even be defined accurately by the ratio of cholesterol to bile salts plus lecithin, because the last two components have differing actions and these are not additive [4]. (On the other hand, the reserve cholesterol-dissolving capacity of an undersaturated bile can be expressed in terms of how much extra cholesterol can be dissolved in it. This attractively direct approach has been used surprisingly little, but is currently being explored [321, 322]). A dilute bile can be supersaturated with cholesterol as easily as a strong one, if not more so.

To express pictorially the composition of a three-membered mixture it is easiest and clearest to use triangular co-ordinates (Fig. 3.15). The same triangle can be used as a phase diagram, since the physical state of cholesterol in bile seems to be determined only by the proportions of cholesterol, lecithin and bile salts, provided the water content of bile is within the range of 75-96 per cent [4]. In 1968 Admirand & Small applied this technique to samples of gallbladder bile aspirated at laparotomy in patients with cholesterol or mixed gallstones. Their results are shown in Fig. 12.1, which shows a clear separation between

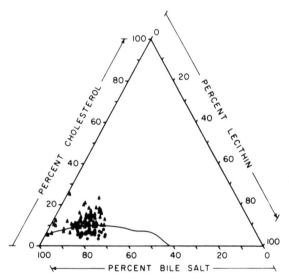

Fig. 12.1. The composition of gallbladder bile, expressed by triangular co-ordinates, from patients with cholesterol or mixed gallstones (triangles) and from controls (circles). The limits of cholesterol solubility, as determined from artificial bile salt-lecithin-cholesterol mixtures, are shown by the curved line. The black triangles represent biles which contained microcrystals of cholesterol, the white triangles those without microcrystals (from Admirand & Small [4]).

controls and gallstone patients. All controls have biles with a composition below the line of maximum cholesterol solubility, that is in the micellar zone. Biles from gallstone patients without microcrystals fall on or very near the line, indicating saturation with cholesterol. Biles from patients with stones and microcrystals are well above the line.

This important study was the first one to show a consistent difference in bile composition between gallstone patients and controls. This fact validates the physicochemical approach to bile so brilliantly developed by Small [603] and also provides a means of identifying lithogenic bile. Further, with this analytical technique, it seems one can predict the future development of cholelithiasis. An investigation of a stone-free population (young South-West American Indian women), with a 70 per cent expectation of developing gallstones within a few years [547], has shown half the subjects to have bile that is already lithogenic, that is predestined to contain stones [656, 680].

Other recent studies have gone a long way towards defining the pathogenesis of this physicochemical lesion. In 1970 two groups of workers confirmed the suggestion of Burnett [81] that the bile of gallstone patients is lithogenic before it enters the gallbladder. Using triangular co-ordinates, Vlahcevic et al. [681] found the composition of hepatic bile to be essentially the same as that of gallbladder bile from the same subject, while Small & Rapo [608] found that on average gallbladder bile was right on the limiting line of cholesterol solubility and hepatic bile was over the line. Despite this minor disagreement, these studies undoubtedly end the long argument as to the role of the gallbladder in the production of lithogenic bile. It can now be stated that the gallbladder is merely the innocent victim of a delinquent liver, being the relatively quiet backwater where crystal nucleation and growth can take place.

The basis of gallstone disease is therefore the secretion by the liver of bile containing an excess of cholesterol in relation to its solvents, bile salts and phospholipid (lecithin). Such an abnormality could arise from the secretion of an absolute excess of cholesterol or from the secretion of amounts of bile salt and/or lecithin which are inadequate to dissolve a normal load of cholesterol. Ideally the distinction would be made by measurements of total daily secretion of the three components in patients with gallstones and in controls. Unfortunately such measurements depend on continuous access to the common bile duct, and can therefore be made only in patients with T-tube drainage, who inevitably have undergone cholecystectomy or have an otherwise abnormal biliary system. Analysis of tube-aspirated duodenal contents suggests that gallstone patients do not secrete excessive quantities of cholesterol but do secrete subnormal quantities of lecithin [637]. Since lecithin secretion is largely dependent on bile salt secretion (see Chapter 8) this implies deficient secretion of bile salts.

The vast majority of secreted bile salts are recirculated rather than newly synthesised. Hence, the main determinant of bile salt secretion is the size of the circulating pool. It has recently been shown by Vlahcevic et al. [679] that the total bile salt pool is reduced to 1.29 g, or little more than half normal, in men with gallstones present in radiologically functioning gallbladders. In unpublished studies we have found a similar reduction in women with gallstones. It could be argued that the reduced pool is the result rather than the cause of the gallstones. However, reduced pool sizes have also been reported in young U.S. Indian women with a high probability of developing cholelithiasis but with as yet normal gallbladders [680].

Thus it seems very likely that the basis of lithogenic bile is a reduced bile salt pool size. Indeed, Vlahcevic et al. have shown that subjects who secrete supersaturated bile have a significantly reduced bile salt pool [30a, 680], and have suggested a critical level of 1.6-1.8 g [637]. The aetiology of the reduced bile salt pool is discussed on page 156.

The above findings explain many earlier reports that the ratios bile salts/cholesterol and lecithin/cholesterol are on average lower in the gallbladder bile of gallstone patients than controls (for references see Admirand & Small [4]).

OTHER BILE SALT ALTERATIONS IN CHOLELITHIASIS

As Van der Linden has pointed out [674], in all recent studies in which the bile of gallstone patients has been compared with controls, there has been a lower trihydroxy to dihydroxy bile acid ratio in stone-bearing bile (though this does not apply to the recent study of Thistle & Schoenfield [656]). This change is due to an increased proportion of deoxycholate [81, 469], and there is some evidence of increased lithocholate also [469]. The increased bacterial alteration of bile salts which these changes imply has not been explained. It may be due to gallbladder dysfunction, since a similar increase in deoxycholate has been noted after cholecystectomy (see Chapter 14). Bacterial infection of the biliary tract is unlikely to be the explanation [81].

It has been speculated that relative excess of dihydroxy bile salts may be lithogenic, on the grounds that the dihydroxy micelle is less polar and so less stable than the trihydroxy one [647]. On the other hand, dihydroxy bile salts, and especially deoxycholates [162], have a superior capacity for solubilising cholesterol (though the difference from trihydroxy salts is minimised by the presence of lecithin) [286]. In any case a low tri-OH/di-OH ratio is seen in patients with pigment stones [336], which supports the idea that it is a result of the gallstones, not a cause.

The glycine/taurine conjugation ratio has been said to be slightly reduced in gallstone patients [81] but this has not been confirmed [115]. Glycine conjugates are more efficient at solubilising cholesterol than taurine conjugates [162, 286], but again the difference is minimised with increasing concentrations of lecithin [286].

BILE ACIDS IN GALLSTONES

Bile acids are found in minute quantities in cholesterol-rich stones [336, 468] but can be important constituents of pigment-calcium stones [468]. The bile acids found are the same as those present in bile, except that traces of two ketonic bile acids have been detected (7-ketolithocholic and 12-ketolithocholic) [571]. Schoenfield et al. found traces of free bile acids, while lithocholate was sometimes present in the centres of stones [571]. These workers also reported that in the centres of stones there was an increase in the G/T ratio and a reduction in deoxycholate, and interpreted this as pointing to an interruption of the enterohepatic circulation at the moment of stone genesis. However, Nakayama [468] found no such reduction of deoxycholate; in the stone as a whole there was actually an increase in deoxycholate [469].

The significance of bile acids in the genesis of calcium-pigment gallstones has not been investigated extensively.

EXPERIMENTAL CHOLELITHIASIS

Full reviews of this subject have recently appeared [65, 621] and it will only be mentioned briefly here under four headings. The main situations where bile salts are involved are:

(1) *Lithocholate feeding* combined with a low protein diet induces stones to form in the common duct of rats (see page 123).

(2) *Cholestanol* (or dehydrocholesterol) 0.25-1.0 per cent in the diet of rabbits causes them to form gallstones composed mainly of the glycine conjugate of allodeoxycholic acid [311]. This animal model provides an elegant demonstration of bile acid metabolism and physical chemistry [304] and is attractive to the investigator [65], but it has no known relevance to human cholelithiasis.

(3) *Cholestyramine* 1 per cent in the diet of weight-losing guinea-pigs caused most of them to form stones containing 50 per cent cholesterol, and at the same time the ratio of bile acids to cholesterol in the bile fell [569]. However, in hamsters cholestyramine 3 per cent in the diet prevented or abolished gallstones induced by a high sugar, fat-free diet [33] and increased the bile acid/cholesterol ratio [35], while in mice it had no effect [34]. It should be added that in man cholestyramine has an indefinite effect on the bile acid/cholesterol ratio [675].

(4) *High glucose or sucrose, fat-free and fibre-free diets* regularly produce cholesterol-rich gallstones in hamsters, together with a fall in the biliary bile salt concentration and a rise in the cholesterol concentration [113, 295]. These effects are reduced or abolished by substituting uncooked starch for the sugar, by adding bulk-forming agents such as carboxymethyl cellulose, and by adding fat, especially if it is rich in polyunsaturated fatty acids [113, 295]. Of all animal models this is clearly the most relevant to the problem of human cholelithiasis, and it has been extensively discussed from this viewpoint [113, 295]. Its relevance is increased by the fact that animals on this diet also develop diabetes [295], since there is a definite clinical association between gallstones and diabetes.

THE AETIOLOGY OF HUMAN GALLSTONES: THE REFINING OF DIETARY CARBOHYDRATE?

Recent investigations have revealed that many apparently normal Swedes [469], Danes [116] and U.S. Indians [656, 680] secrete bile that is supersaturated with cholesterol. If it is accepted that a bile salt pool size of under 1.8 g is lithogenic [637], then 30 per cent of U.S. white males secrete abnormal bile [684]. A recent survey in the Bristol area of England has shown a threefold rise in the annual rate of gallbladder operations since 1940. Why has this metabolic disease* become so common in Western countries? The writer believes that current knowledge of bile acid and cholesterol metabolism is such that a hypothesis can be constructed for gallstone aetiology, which is consistent with the epidemiology of cholelithiasis and with new nutritional concepts of the effects of carbohydrate-refining.

This hypothesis is based on the premise that the essential defect in gallstone disease is impairment of liver synthesis of bile salts. This premise derives from the studies of Vlahcevic *et al.* [30a, 680] in American Indians. These workers have shown that, in both men and women, those who secrete lithogenic bile (whether or not they have actually formed gallstones) have a reduced bile salt pool and yet have a normal daily turnover of bile salts. This normal turnover in the face of a reduced pool is interpreted as meaning that, in spite of being subjected to a maximal stimulus, the liver is unable to increase its synthetic rate.

The following illustration may help to explain this concept (the figures used are based on the data of Bell *et al.* [30a]). A normal subject, with a 2000 mg bile salt pool circulating eight times daily, perfuses his liver with a total of 16 g bile salt each day. He maintains his pool size constant by varying his liver synthesis of new bile salt. According to current concepts of feedback inhibition, it is the 16 g of bile salt returning to the liver which keeps daily synthesis down to the normal 400 mg, this being all that is necessary to replace faecal losses. If the daily return of bile salt is reduced, that is if the enterohepatic circulation is interrupted, then liver synthesis increases. From monkey experiments [154], one would expect a 20 per cent interruption to cause maximal synthesis. A 20 per cent interruption is equivalent to a return of 12.8 g bile salt daily. Therefore, a normal subject should synthesise maximally (approximately 3.3 g/day [94]) if his bile salt return is reduced to 12.8 g/day.

---

* It has often been suggested that bile stasis, produced by fasting or by female hormones, is important but it can hardly play more than a permissive or secondary role, since gallstones are so rare in primitive societies. Infection is also regarded as secondary or unrelated, because of the rarity of acalculous cholecystitis, because most gallstones are asymptomatic, and because many stone-bearing gallbladders are virtually normal.

A man with lithogenic bile has on average a bile salt pool of 1.1 g. Assuming he recycles his pool the normal eight times per day, he perfuses his liver with 8.8 g bile salt daily. In a normal person this would constitute a supra-maximal stimulus to liver synthesis. Nevertheless, the secretor of lithogenic bile synthesises only the normal 400 mg/day. His liver is insensitive or inhibited. Expressed differently, the lithogenic liver is a liver in which cholesterol catabolism is pathologically suppressed.

The Japanese workers at Kyoto have also postulated that cholesterol catabolism is impaired, and have suggested that this is due to deficiency of essential fatty acids (E.F.A.). They believe that cholesterol must be esterified with fatty acid before being catabolised, and that catabolism is slowed down if E.F.A.s such as arachidonic acid are not available for this esterification [295]. They found that adding E.F.A.-rich fats to a high sugar, fat-free diet was more effective than adding saturated fat or oleic acid-rich fat in preventing gallstone formation in hamsters. Also in the livers of gallstone patients only 8 per cent of the fatty acid was arachidonic compared with 11 per cent in controls [168]. Hikasa et al. believe that this E.F.A. deficiency is accentuated by a high intake of saturated fat, especially butter, which interferes with the activation of vitamin B_6 which in turn is necessary for E.F.A. metabolism. In their animal experiments B_6 deficiency was in some circumstances a pre-requisite for stone formation [295]. These workers concede that gallstone patients do not show other evidence of E.F.A. or vitamin B_6 deficiency. They also agree with the extensive experience of Dam [113] that the one essential requirement of a lithogenic diet is that it should contain a great deal of highly available carbohydrate (sucrose, glucose or soluble starch). Addition of raw, insoluble carbohydrate prevents cholelithiasis.

It seems to the present writer that it is unnecessary to invoke E.F.A.s in the pathogenesis of impaired bile acid synthesis/cholesterol catabolism. A sufficient explanation is available in the known effects of diets rich in highly available carbohydrate, that is carbohydrate which has been refined or stripped of fibre, especially if one also considers the known effects of supplementing the diet with cellulose or artificial bulk-forming agents.

It has been repeatedly shown in both rats [256, 525] and rabbits [293] that on semi-synthetic, low-residue diets containing a high proportion of sugar or processed starch, bile acid turnover is lower than on ordinary or natural food. Likewise, African Negroes placed on a low-residue diet excreted less bile acids than they did on their normal high-roughage diet [10]. Conversely, adding roughage to the diet in the form of powdered cellulose (to make up 20 per cent of the diet) greatly increased bile acid turnover in rats on a refined diet [525, 632], and increased bile acid excretion in young girls on a hypercholesterolaemic regime [584]. Similarly, addition of an artificial bulk-forming agent (psyllium hydrocolloid or Metamucil) to the diet markedly increased bile acid excretion rates in young men [194] and in rats [28]. Thus there is little doubt that consumption of refined, fibre-depleted diets is a possible cause of impaired bile acid synthesis and cholesterol catabolism.

The relevance of these findings to gallstones is increased by the fact that when the size of the bile salt pool has been measured in rats on such refined diets it has been found to be reduced to half normal [380, 524, 525]. Adding cellulose or Metamucil to the diet expands the pool [28, 525].

The effects of refined and unrefined diets on the size of the bile salt pool and on biliary lipid composition in man have not been reported, and will clearly be of great importance to the present hypothesis.* However, it has been reported that the American Indians who have such a strong propensity for forming lithogenic bile with a small bile salt pool [680] subsist largely on refined carbohydrate [369].

The mechanism whereby refined carbohydrate inhibits bile salt synthesis remains to be worked out, but two possibilities deserve to be discussed. These are the toxicity of absorbed lithocholic acid and a change in lipid metabolism consequent on excessively rapid carbohydrate absorption.

There are good theoretical grounds for expecting lithocholate to be absorbed more than normal on a refined carbohydrate diet. These are (a) less dietary fibre means less solid residue in the bowel lumen to which lithocholate can adsorb; and (b) the slower intestinal transit and more concentrated bowel contents which result from a low-fibre diet increase the chances of lithocholate making contact with the gut mucosa. Having been absorbed, lithocholate is capable of inhibiting bile salt synthesis by its effect on microsomal 12α-hydroxylation [466]. It is well established that lithocholate increases liver cholesterol levels [328, 389, 466]. It remains to be seen whether it influences biliary bile salt/cholesterol ratios.

* Such studies are in progress in the author's laboratory.

The concept that rapid absorption of readily available carbohydrate may influence cholesterol catabolism has no direct experimental support except the 1934 report of Wright & Whipple [711] that feeding sugar to bile fistula dogs caused a sharper drop in bile salt excretion than in cholesterol excretion. However, it is in harmony with recent work linking diet-induced hyperinsulinism with abnormal cholesterol metabolism [626, 627]. Also Sarles et al. have reported that, in patients with T-tubes after biliary surgery, the bile cholesterol concentration rises with a high calorie intake [552]. Sarles et al. have also shown by dietary surveys that on average gallstone patients take in more calories than controls [550]. It is common experience and common logic that the dietary component most likely to cause chronic over-consumption of calories is refined carbohydrate, due to the fact that carbohydrate foods as commonly taken are in an artificially concentrated form (sucrose and sucrose-enriched bakeries, confectionery etc.).

There are other grounds besides experimental data for relating cholelithiasis to the consumption of refined carbohydrate, namely the epidemiology and clinical associations of gallstones.

Cholelithiasis is one of a group of diseases whose incidence in different countries parallels the degree of economic development. Like obesity, diabetes, coronary artery disease, diverticular disease and cancer of the colon, cholelithiasis is rare in tribal Africans, but increasingly common in American Negroes. It probably diminished in incidence in Europe in the 1939-1945 war, but has certainly become commoner since. It has also increased rapidly in the urban Japanese. These changes in incidence have been paralleled by changes in carbohydrate consumption. With increasing affluence there is always a reduction in intake of relatively unrefined cereals and a sharp increase in intake of sugar (and animal fat). Total fibre intake decreases substantially, which probably explains the altered colon function leading to diverticular disease [103, 498] as well as the increase in colon cancer [79]. At the same time, consumption of artificially concentrated carbohydrate foods, especially those based on sugar and white flour, leads to obesity and diabetes and is probably a major determinant of coronary artery disease [103]. Clinically there are associations between gallstones and obesity, gallstones and diabetes, gallstones and coronary artery disease, obesity and diabetes, obesity and coronary disease, and diabetes and coronary disease. The more closely patients with one of these four diseases are examined the more they are found to have features of the other three. This closely spun web of associations strongly suggests that all four diseases have a common aetiology. The only hypothesis known to the author which fits all these facts is that elaborated by Cleave in a joint work [103], namely that all these diseases are caused by eating refined carbohydrate.

The effect of diet on bile salt and cholesterol metabolism is discussed further in Chapter 16.

THE ROLE OF BACTERIAL INFECTION

Although bacterial infection is now discounted as the primary cause of cholesterol-rich gallstones, mechanisms have been established whereby biliary infection could contribute to stone formation. In particular deconjugation of bile salts could be followed by diffusion of free bile acids out of the gallbladder [495] resulting in a falling bile salt/cholesterol ratio. Alternatively, bacteria possessing the enzyme phospholipase A may split lecithin to lysolecithin and fatty acid. If the fatty acid were then absorbed, as it can be by the guinea-pig gallbladder [473], there would be a loss of detergent power [474] and possibly precipitation of cholesterol. (The same sequence could follow reflux of pancreatic juice which contains phospholipase A.)

The common pigment stone of the Far East consists mainly of insoluble calcium bilirubinate and probably derives from bacterial hydrolysis of conjugated bilirubin by the β-glucuronidase present in E. coli [602]. This process could also be important in providing a pigment nucleus (seeding agent) round which cholesterol could crystallise from super-saturated bile in the initiation and growth of cholesterol-rich gallstones. However, cholesterol does not require a pigment nucleus for crystallisation to occur [633]. In any case it is clear that the primary defect in Western gallstone disease is secretion of lithogenic bile.

In the unusual event of acalculous cholecystitis, the damaged gallbladder wall can probably absorb bile salts. Conceivably this could lead to stone formation. On the other hand Izumi [336] found bile lipid relationships to be normal in patients with acalculous cholecystitis.

The role of mucus is not discounted here, but clearly a sticking agent can only be active if there are particles for it to stick together.

UNUSUAL CAUSES OF CHOLELITHIASIS

In *cirrhosis of the liver* there is a two- to threefold increase in the incidence of gallstones [63]. This may be because the size of the bile salt pool is reduced [683], but the lipid composition of the bile has not been reported.

In *resection and disease of the terminal ileum* the incidence of gallstones is increased four- or fivefold [105, 285]. Again this may be due to bile salt deficiency. In two suitably studied cases the bile was found to be saturated with cholesterol [105]. Theoretically, increased production of lithocholate in the colon could lead to calcium glycolithocholate precipitating in the bile [602], but analysis of stones and bile from two patients revealed no lithocholic acid [105].

CHOLECYSTITIS

If it is accepted that cholecystitis is generally secondary to cholelithiasis then it can be regarded as a bile salt related disease. The actual pathogenesis of cholecystitis is poorly understood. Direct bacterial invasion is seldom the cause, but bacterial deconjugation of bile salts could perhaps play a role, since free bile salts and especially deoxycholate are strongly toxic to the gallbladder wall of dogs [8]. There is also evidence to incriminate lysolecithin, the hydrolytic breakdown product of lecithin. It has been found in inflamed human gallbladders and can produce cholecystitis in rabbits [232].

Once the gallbladder wall is damaged there may, as mentioned above, be abnormal absorption of bile salts. In mice this can lead to the bile becoming lithogenic [83], but there is evidence against this being a significant factor in man [336].

DISSOLUTION OF GALLSTONES

Gallstones can be dissolved not only by being placed in a dog's gallbladder but also by being incubated *in vitro* with bile salt-lecithin mixtures, and to a lesser extent with pure bile salt solutions [97, 162].

In vivo it is possible by feeding chenodeoxycholic acid to restore lithogenic bile to normal, due to an expansion of the bile salt pool [656], and it has recently been reported that this treatment caused gallstones to disappear or decrease in size in four out of seven patients [127]. However, such treatment must be regarded as experimental in view of a number of possible hazards [605]. In particular, the suppression of endogenous bile salt synthesis which must occur may, unless cholesterol synthesis is equally suppressed, result in accumulation of cholesterol within the body.

Feeding phospholipids has been reported to increase biliary phospholipid levels [664], but this claim has been disputed [655]. It is to be hoped that this controversy will soon be settled by controlled trials on adequate numbers of subjects having an intact enterohepatic circulation. A positive effect would be hard to reconcile with the reported failure of orally administered radioactive lecithin to appear intact in the bile [554].

13 Diseases in which Bile Salts may be Important

PANCREATITIS (ACUTE HAEMORRHAGIC)

Many theories have been advanced for the pathogenesis of pancreatitis, of which the most durable is the bile reflux hypothesis. The evidence that bile can flow from the common bile duct to the pancreas, and that bile in the pancreas is toxic, has been extensively reviewed [266]. There is also evidence that duodenal contents (which may, of course, be bile-rich) can reflux into the pancreatic duct [417].When Pure bile salt solutions are injected into the pancreatic duct of animals they induce all grades of inflammation and necrosis up to acute haemorrhagic pancreatitis. In rats, free bile salts are about twice as toxic as conjugates, and di-hydroxy bile salts are four to eight times more toxic than cholates, as judged by the concentrations necessary to produce pancreatitis [266]. Hansson found excess di-hydroxy bile salts, mainly chenodeoxycholate, in the bile of seven out of nine patients with acute pancreatitis but this could be due to coincidental liver dysfunction [266]. He also found free bile acids in the bile of three and in the duodenal contents of seven out of 45 patients with acute pancreatitis, but their significance is speculative.

The mode of action of bile salts in damaging the pancreas is attracting considerable attention. Beck *et al.* [27] found that a synthetic anionic detergent, lauryl sulphate, produced lesions in the dog pancreas which were morphologically similar to those produced by bile salts, suggesting that the latter act through their detergency. On the other hand, Schmidt & Creutzfeldt [566] have postulated that bile salts act by activating the pancreatic enzyme phospholipase A which converts lecithin to lysolecithin, and that it is lysolecithin which actually damages the pancreas. Certainly lysolecithin can be detected in the pancreas of patients who have died of acute pancreatitis [566] and in the gland of rats given bile salts into the pancreatic duct [15].

It is only fair to add that some workers doubt that bile reflux is involved in the pathogenesis of acute pancreatitis, and prefer to stress the role of proteases, elastase and kinins [110, 417].

GASTRITIS AND GASTRIC ULCER

These two conditions are discussed together because gastritis is invariably present to some degree in patients with gastric ulcer. Indeed current thinking is that gastritis is the primary lesion [218] and that the ulcer arises in that part of the gastritic or 'alkaline' area which is nearest to acid-secreting mucosa [487]. This and the fact of 'no ulcer, no acid' implicate acid-pepsin secretion in the pathogenesis. However, acid alone cannot be responsible for ulcer formation, since the acid-secreting capacity of the stomach is on average less than normal in gastric ulcer patients. Therefore an additional factor must operate. The two main candidates are gastric stasis and bile reflux. The cases for and against the stasis and reflux hypotheses have been lucidly discussed in a very recent and well documented article by Rhodes [531]. One of the best pieces of evidence for reflux is the demonstration by Rhodes himself and his co-workers of high bile salt concentrations (mean 5.3 mM) in the post-prandial gastric juice of ulcer patients [532].

A key part of the bile reflux hypothesis is the toxicity of bile for the gastric mucosa. This toxicity has been demonstrated in three ways. (1) Gastritis has been produced in dogs and rats by diverting bile into the stomach or perfusing it into gastric pouches [531]. Actual ulceration may occur [361, 613] and, if there is repeated exposure to bile, atrophic gastritis is produced [531]. (2) Bile alters free gastric mucus from a white viscous material into a transparent one in which all the epithelial cells have been lysed [236]. Adherent mucus is depleted [531]. (3) Bile breaks the gastric mucosal barrier which normally prevents back-diffusion of hydrogen ions into the mucosa. The precise nature of this barrier is uncertain. It may be mucus or the lipoprotein cell membrane of epithelial cells. It is normally weakest in the antrum, which is the main site of gastric ulcers [332], and it is breached by known gastro-toxic agents such as aspirin. In patients with gastritis and gastric ulcer there is abnormal permeability of the mucosa to acid, that is, a weakened barrier, which may well explain the apparent hyposecretion of acid in these subjects [497].

Breaching of the mucosal barrier is associated with a fall in the potential difference across the mucosa [217], and such a fall has been demonstrated with exposure of the mucosa to bile-rich duodenal contents [217] and to pure bile [47]. Black et al. [47] have made the important observation that the action of bile is greater at lower pH values. This suggests that it is acid which actually damages the mucosa, but that bile is necessary to make the mucosa permeable and therefore vulnerable to the acid. This concept agrees with the fact that gastric mucosa is not damaged by being implanted in the gallbladder [531] and explains the 'no acid, no ulcer' axiom.

The effect of pure bile salts in breaching this barrier was first shown in dogs [131] but has now been demonstrated in man also. Thus Ivey et al. [334] found that a 5.5 mM solution of taurine-conjugated bile salts (84 per cent taurocholate) reversed the direction of movement of H^+ and Cl^- ions across the human stomach when it was instilled with 160 mM hydrochloric acid. The loss of H^+ ions from the lumen was roughly balanced by a gain of Na^+ ions—further evidence of a leaky mucosa. At the same time a significant absorption of bile salts took place from the stomach [333] (as also occurs in the dog [130]). Pure glycine-conjugated bile salts have not yet been studied in this way but it is likely that they would be absorbed better than taurine conjugates since at pH 1-2 they are almost wholly non-ionised. On the other hand they are also precipitated at this pH, so it is hard to predict whether glycine conjugates would be more or less gastro-toxic than taurine conjugates in vivo.

If bile salts are involved in the genesis of gastric ulcer, their effects should be antagonised by carbenoxolone, the one drug which definitely promotes ulcer healing. Rhodes and his co-workers have in fact shown that pre-treatment of dog gastric pouches with carbenoxolone greatly reduces the damaging effect of bile [531]. This is particularly relevant since carbenoxolone is already known to stimulate mucus secretion by gastric epithelial cells, as well as to prolong their life span [406]. The intriguing picture that this evokes is of bile and carbenoxolone doing battle over the question of whether the giant HCl should be allowed to penetrate mucosa intacta. However, the effect of carbenoxolone is a non-specific one [406] and its therapeutic value cannot be used as an argument for bile salts being the damaging agent.

In their examination of the bile reflux hypothesis, Rhodes and his co-workers have looked at the effect of cholestyramine on healing, and of healing itself on bile reflux. In a controlled trial, cholestyramine-treated patients had a greater mean reduction in ulcer size, but the difference did not reach statistical significance (possibly because cholestyramine is emptied from the stomach with the meal) [531]. In their other study they showed no consistent change in intra-gastric bile salt concentrations after ulcers had healed [48]. This proves no more than that the ulcer does not cause the reflux, but suggests that other factors besides bile aggression are involved in ulcerogenesis. These other factors are probably related to mucosal resistance. For example stress, as in haemorrhagic shock, impairs mucosal permeability [601], possibly through the inhibitory actions of adrenaline and corticosteroids on mucus production and on the replication of epithelial cells [406].

The bile reflux hypothesis is consistent with a possible role for lysolecithin, which is certainly capable of damaging the stomach [132]. Production of lysolecithin from the lecithin in bile and food is aided by the action of bile salts in activating pancreatic phospholipase A [566].

In certain circumstances, drugs such as aspirin and alcohol may also be involved in the genesis of gastritis and gastric ulcer. This discussion does not seek to be a complete review of gastric ulcer aetiology.

TROPICAL SPRUE

In spite of much work the nature of this disease remains an enigma. The common occurrence of fat and vitamin B_{12} malabsorption together with the therapeutic effect of antibiotics suggests the presence of bacterial overgrowth in the small intestine [224]. Recent bacteriological studies have in fact shown that there is always an abnormal flora in the upper small bowel, often including enteric bacteria. However, there is overlap with the findings in malnourished but otherwise well individuals, which suggests the presence of other factors in tropical sprue, possibly host resistance [224].

Studies of bile salt metabolism have added a little to our understanding of this disease. Firstly, two groups of workers have shown that there is no excessive deconjugation of bile salts in the small intestine [98, 348]. This shows that the steatorrhoea is different in origin from that occurring in the stagnant loop syndrome. Secondly, there is preliminary evidence that the turnover rate of cholic acid may be moderately increased [670]. This would be consistent with mild bile salt malabsorption due to involvement of the terminal ileum by the non-specific mucosal abnormality, as would the usual defect in vitamin B_{12} absorption. It is unlikely that mild bile salt malabsorption would affect the bile salt pool size. Nevertheless, a reduction in post-prandial bile salt concentrations in the jejunum has been reported by one group [670] (but not by another [98]). If this finding is confirmed, it may be explained by impaired gallbladder emptying as noted in coeliac disease (see below), which would also mask any tendency to malabsorption of bile salts. It is possible therefore that steatorrhoea in this disease is contributed to by intraluminal bile salt deficiency.

Abnormalities in the composition of the bile salt pool have been reported, but the situation is not yet clear. In Vellore, S. India, the G/T ratio was significantly higher in eight sprue patients than in six controls [347], whereas in West Bengal the G/T ratio in three sprue patients was very low [464]. Two other unexplained findings were made by the latter group, reduction or absence of glycochenodeoxycholate and excess of conjugated lithocholate. Further work is necessary.

ADULT COELIAC DISEASE (IDIOPATHIC STEATORRHOEA, NON-TROPICAL SPRUE)

Low-Beer *et al.* [410] studied the recirculation of ring-labelled taurocholate and its metabolites in 11 patients with flat jejunal biopsies. The half-life of taurocholate was prolonged to an average of 3.5 days (control 1.1 days) and in most cases the appearance of labelled metabolites in the bile was delayed. It was thought that these changes were due to impaired gallbladder emptying in response to food, with consequent protection of bile salts from bacterial attack and the risk of excretion, and this was supported by radiological studies. The hypothesis to explain this gallbladder inertia and sluggish circulation of bile salts was impaired release of cholecystokinin by the damaged small bowel mucosa [410]. In this study jejunal bile salt concentrations during digestion were not measured. However, low values were found by Miettinen and Siurala [439] in two out of seven cases, and by other workers in several isolated patients [373, 419, 673]. The amount of digested fat in the micellar phase tends to be low, but lipolysis is probably normal [439] in spite of evidence that pancreozymin stimulation of pancreatic secretion is impaired [150]. Thus it is likely that in some patients with coeliac disease there is intraluminal bile salt deficiency, and this might be a contributing factor in the steatorrhoea of this disease.

The small intestinal flora is usually normal in adult coeliac disease [224], but one case has been reported in which bacterial overgrowth was associated with bile salt deconjugation in the upper small bowel [538].

The bile salt pattern in the bile is generally found to be normal in our laboratory, but Miettinen [439] has reported a tendency to a reduced proportion of deoxycholate.

NON-SPECIFIC DIARRHOEA

In a double-blind study in Boston, long-standing diarrhoea which had been attributed to the irritable colon syndrome was relieved by cholestyramine therapy in five out of 12 patients [558]. Whether this indicates a functional bile salt malabsorption, perhaps due to rapid ileal transit, remains to be seen. The possibility of ileocaecal sphincter incompetence was discussed on page 80. Further reports in the near future are expected. Meanwhile it has been found that cholestyramine does not help in acute tropical diarrhoea in Vietnam [416], nor in ulcerative colitis [436], which suggests that bile salt catharsis is not involved in all varieties of diarrhoea.

CARCINOMA OF THE COLON

In a comparison of faeces from inhabitants of areas with high and low incidences of carcinoma of the colon, Hill et al. [296] noted relatively more anaerobes, and more strains able to 7α-dehydroxylate cholic acid in samples from high incidence areas (England, Scotland, U.S.A.) than from low incidence areas (Uganda, India, rural Japan). Afro-Asian stools also contained relatively few highly degraded bile acids, and (rather surprisingly in view of the well-documented effect of dietary fibre in increasing bile acid excretion) low total concentrations of bile salts. All these changes except the last are explicable by the more rapid intestinal transit which is present in subjects such as Ugandans who eat a great deal of vegetable fibre [79]. However, Hill et *al.* have discussed their findings in terms of dietary fat. More convincingly, they have pointed to the chemical similarity between bile acids and known carcinogens such as methylcholanthrene, and postulated that colonic cancer is caused by excessive exposure of the mucosa to degraded bile salts including deoxycholate. This exposure will be conditional most of all on the rate of stool transit and on stool concentration, both of which are governed by the amount of fibre in the diet [79, 103]. Much work needs to be done to substantiate this interesting and important hypothesis.

In view of the close clinical and epidemiological association between colonic carcinoma and polyps of the colon, as well as with ulcerative colitis [79], it is conceivable that these other two diseases are also responses of the colon to excessively concentrated or abnormally degraded bile salts.

HYPERCHOLESTEROLAEMIA

Since bile salt synthesis and excretion account for nearly half of cholesterol turnover (see Chapter 8), diminished bile salt turnover could well result in accumulation of cholesterol in the body. Despite the obvious importance of this point there have been few comparisons of bile salt turnover in normal and hypercholesterolaemic subjects. The marked person-to-person variation in bile salt turnover (Table 7.1) makes it difficult to show group differences of moderate degree. Nevertheless there is considerable evidence in the literature that in essential hypercholesterolaemia (type II hyperlipoproteinaemia) bile salt turnover is reduced. Thus Miettinen *et al.* [437] found the mean daily faecal excretion of bile acids to be 220 mg in control subjects and only 154 mg in eight siblings with familial hypercholesterolaemia. Recently, Grundy *et al.* [248] found the average bile acid excretion in nine American patients with type II hyperlipoproteinaemia to be 225 mg/day. This is distinctly lower than the values found in normal Americans in other investigations [18, 108, 447]. Similarly, turnover studies using labelled cholic acid have shown a tendency towards reduced turnover in essential hypercholesterolaemia (90 mg daily in two patients [401]; 161-191 mg/day in four patients, compared with 295-314 mg/day in nine normal subjects [289]). The data of Hellström & Lindstedt [289] and of Austad [16] suggest that this is due to a prolonged half-life rather than a reduced pool size of cholic acid. It has been noted on several occasions that the bile of hypercholesterolaemic patients contains subnormal amounts of deoxycholate [289]. Since deoxycholate is formed in the colon, this finding suggests decreased entry of bile salts into the colon (or less probably reduced ability of colonic bacteria to dehydroxylate cholic acid or impaired absorption of deoxycholate from the colon). Reduced entry of bile salts into the colon implies over-efficient absorption of bile salts in the small intestine. The latter phenomenon would explain the prolonged cholate half-life and the reduced faecal excretion of bile salts mentioned above.

The hypothesis is advanced, therefore, that 'essential hypercholesterolaemia' is, at least in some cases, a defect of small intestinal function leading to over-efficient ileal absorption of bile salts. As to the nature of this defect, the possibilities include abnormally slow passage of intestinal contents through the ileum, and reduced volume of ileal contents due to excessive fluid absorption more proximally.

In Western societies the problem of familial hypercholesterolaemia (type II hyperlipoproteinaemia) is overshadowed by the much greater question of why the 'normal range' of serum cholesterol is so high, in comparison with countries like Japan and Africa where coronary artery disease is still as rare as it was in England 50 years ago. The answer may again be over-efficient ileal absorption of bile salts but due this time to dietary factors. Nutritionists agree that the greatest change in the English diet in the last century has been the reduction in consumption of relatively unrefined cereal foods (brown bread, oats, etc.) which contain fibre, and the increased consumption of fibre-free foods containing sugar and to a lesser extent white flour. The increase in fat intake is small by comparison [103, 133].

Primitive diets are generally rich in fibre. As discussed on pages 70 and 190, dietary fibre promotes bile salt excretion, probably by increasing the volume and transit rate of intestinal contents. In subjects eating fibre-free liquid formula diets, deoxycholate tends to disappear from the bile [402]. Animals on similar diets have reduced bile salt excretion [293, 525]. It is possible therefore that a major determinant of blood cholesterol levels is the amount of bile salt carried into the colon and this is determined by the amount of fibre in the diet. There is considerable evidence that a high fibre intake does lower serum cholesterol [584, 666]. This hypothesis is essentially the same as that developed in relation to gallstones in Chapter 12, which includes clinical and epidemiological evidence (see also Chapter 16).

The biochemical defect appears to be quite different when there is marked hypertriglyceridaemia as well as hypercholesterolaemia. Kottke [367] found the total bile salt synthesis rate to be much higher (mean 1094 mg/day) than it is in simple hypercholesterolaemia (282 mg/day). Similarly Grundy & Ahrens [244] found low bile salt excretion rates in type II hyperlipoproteinaemia but normal or high rates in two patients with the type V defect.

The hypercholesterolaemia of hypothyroidism may be due to a relatively greater inhibition of bile acid synthesis than of cholesterol synthesis [125] (see page 175).

Essential hypercholesterolaemia, or type II hyperlipoproteinaemia, may be effectively treated by interrupting the enterohepatic circulation. This can be done either by cholestyramine therapy or by surgical bypass of the terminal ileum. In both cases there is increased faecal excretion of bile acids (see Chapters 10 and 15). This drain on the body cholesterol pool is only partly balanced by increased cholesterol synthesis, so that the pool size diminishes, the plasma level falls and xanthomas shrink [76, 449, 615]. It is unproved but likely that the progress of atherosclerosis is halted [76, 615].

DISSEMINATED SCLEROSIS

Naqvi et al. [471] recently made the provocative observation that lithocholic acid was present in the diseased brain tissue of a patient who had died with multiple sclerosis, but not in a control brain. Since the same workers have also found lithocholate in the brains of guinea-pigs with experimental allergic encephalomyelitis [470], it is reasonable to suspect that lithocholate may be involved in the pathogenesis of demyelinating diseases. Clearly more data are needed, but in the meantime it is hard to accept the theory of Naqvi et al. [471] that the lithocholate was synthesised by the brain tissue. It seems more likely that it was absorbed from the colon and became adsorbed to the brain. Multiple sclerosis has a similar geographical incidence to cholelithiasis and it is tempting to speculate that its frequency in Western countries is due to a diet-related over-absorption of lithocholate as discussed in relation to gallstone aetiology (page 159).

14 Conditions in which Bile Salt Metabolism is Altered but without Important Pathological Sequelae

ACUTE HEPATITIS

Since cholestasis is an integral part of all but anicteric cases of viral hepatitis, it is not surprising that patients with this disease have high serum bile salt concentrations, especially in the first week or 10 days [88]. In the experience of Carey [88] serum bile salt tends to return to normal before serum bilirubin. In contrast Frosch & Wagener [204] claimed that serum bile salt concentrations remained abnormal longer than conventional liver function tests and advocated their measurement as a superior test. Cronholm et al. [111] merely noted that serum bile acid increases proportionately more than serum bilirubin. The greater simplicity of ordinary tests makes it unlikely that serum bile salts will ever be measured routinely in hepatitis.

The liver in acute hepatitis has difficulty in removing bile salts from the blood, as evidenced by delayed clearance of intravenously injected cholic acid [343, 653]. That there is also difficulty in secreting bile salts into the intestine has long been accepted as the cause of steatorrhoea in hepatitis, but it has only recently been demonstrated that intestinal bile salt concentrations are low during digestion [443]. There are also reduced levels of lipid in the aqueous phase, especially in the presence of steatorrhoea [443].

There are limited data suggesting that the size of the bile salt pool is reduced [653], presumably because of impaired synthesis.

CHOLECYSTECTOMY

The function of the gallbladder is to prepare a store of concentrated detergent ready for immediate use when food is taken (see page 62). Leaving aside the disputed 'post-cholecystectomy syndrome', no serious clinical effects follow removal of the gallbladder, nor would they be expected since some mammalian species such as the rat do not possess a gallbladder. No significant malabsorption occurs, as judged by the relatively crude criterion of faecal fat excretion [372], and jejunal contents during digestion contain normal amounts of lipid in the micellar phase [66]. This suggests that the size of the bile salt pool is not severely reduced by the lack of a storage place. Indeed, in the author's laboratory, isotope studies have shown no obvious difference between total bile salt pool sizes in cholecystectomised women and matched controls [517]* (unlike similar studies in hyperlipidaemic patients [707] and in dogs [706]). Even if the pool size is preserved there may be a lowering of the bile salt concentrations in the small bowel, at least in the early stages of digestion, since the pool is presumably at all times distributed around the organs of the enterohepatic circulation. In the rat, 70 per cent of the pool is present in the small intestine and 25 per cent in the large bowel [38].

Continuous exposure of bile salts to the intestine leads to greater bacterial alteration. We have obtained evidence that in the absence of the gallbladder the rate of deconjugation and dehydroxylation is increased, since transfer of radioactivity from labelled taurocholate to circulating glycine conjugates and to deoxycholates is accelerated [517]. Furthermore the bile of cholecystectomy patients contains relatively twice as much deoxycholate as control subjects [517]. The altered bile acids seem to be efficiently reabsorbed since the rate of loss of radioactivity from the bile is not increased in the absence of a gallbladder. If this finding is generally applicable, it suggests that bile salt absorption is not interfered with by increased exposure to intestinal bacteria, as present in the stagnant loop syndrome. This concept is in harmony with the fact that the rabbit, which circulates almost all its bile salts in dehydroxylated form (glycodeoxycholate), has a prolonged deoxycholate half-life [292]. Both rabbits and patients with the stagnant loop syndrome have high serum bile salt levels but the

* The bile salt pool size in the gallbladder-less rat is approximately 100 mg/kg body weight [29, 38], whereas in the hamster and gerbil (which do have gallbladders) it is about 23 mg and 95 mg/kg respectively [29].

situation in cholecystectomy patients is unknown. The presence or absence of pruritus seems to be no guide.

It may be significant that in the rat, which is the only animal lacking a gallbladder to have had its bile salt metabolism thoroughly investigated, the liver has evolved the ability to re-hydroxylate deoxycholate and lithocholate. If this is a protective response to absorption of large amounts of dehydroxylated bile acids, the question arises whether removal of the gallbladder could be harmful in species like man which lack this hepatic function.

COLECTOMY AND ILEOSTOMY

In subjects with an ileostomy there is a marked reduction in bacterial alteration of bile salts. In the bile this is evident as very low or absent levels of conjugated deoxycholate [438, 454, 507, 508] and by minimal transfer of radioactivity from labelled taurocholate to the di-hydroxy fraction of the bile salt pool [454]. Similar but less marked changes occur in subjects with ileorectal anastomosis [438, 454]. Even more striking changes are present in ileostomy effluent, which contains virtually no bile acids which have been altered beyond simple deconjugation [438, 507, 508]. This cannot be attributed to absence of contact between bile salts and faecal type bacteria because ileostomy effluent does contain considerable numbers of bacteroides and other anaerobes [225, 507]. However, according to Percy-Robb et al. [507], the anaerobic bacteria in ileostomy effluent are unable to dehydroxylate cholic acid in vitro. An additional factor is that, gram for gram, faeces contain 40-50 times more anaerobes than ileostomy effluent [225] and of course the duration of bile salt-microbe contact is much greater with an intact colon.

These changes have no known adverse effect. The rate of turnover of bile salts is normal as judged both by the quantity of bile salt excreted [438, 508] and by the rate of loss of radioactivity from the bile [454]. Dietary fat is digested and absorbed normally [438, 454] and there is probably no excess incidence of gallstones [454].

ENDOCRINE DISEASES

In hypothyroidism there is a raised G/T ratio in the bile of most but not all patients [288, 291, 596]. Cholic acid turnover is somewhat reduced, probably because the half-life is prolonged to a mean of 3.8 days [288]. These changes are reversed by replacement therapy [288, 291]. The low bile salt turnover may well be due to slow intestinal transit and it could be a contributing factor in the hypercholesterolaemia of hypothyroidism [125, 288]. The cause of the high G/T ratio is uncertain. It is reversed by taurine feeding [291] as well as by thyroxine [288]. In rats, experimental hypothyroidism caused a fall in bile salt synthesis and pool size when these were measured by the bile fistula technique [179], but not when they were studied by isotope techniques in the intact animal [629]; the ratio of cholate to chenodeoxycholate in the bile increased [179, 628].

In hyperthyroidism cholic acid turns over more rapidly (mean *T½* 2.1 days) than normal, but it is not clear whether the amount turned over is increased [288]. There is a slight tendency towards an increased proportion of chenodeoxycholic acid in the bile [288]. In rats fed thyroid hormone the chenodeoxycholate/cholate ratio rises greatly [179, 396, 628], due to a rise in the chenodeoxycholate pool [629]. This may be due to the inhibitory effect of thyroid hormone on the 12α-hydroxylation step in bile salt synthesis [37]. Paradoxically the *T½* is unaffected but overall bile salt synthesis increases 50-60 per cent [629].

In growth hormone deficiency there is a predominance of taurine conjugates and probably a reduced bile salt pool size, since the jejunal bile salt concentration is low during digestion. These changes are reversed by treatment with human growth hormone, and there is a particularly marked rise in jejunal concentrations of chenodeoxycholic acid [516]. In hypophysectomised rats a reduction in chenodeoxycholate has been noted [366].

In rats, adrenal insufficiency increases the G/T ratio [294], in rabbits cortisone increases bile acid secretion from the isolated perfused liver [456], and in dogs treatment with adrenaline and nor-adrenaline shortens bile salt half-lives and decreases pool sizes [210], but there are no clinical correlates of these experiments.

15 Bile Salt-binding Agents

Bile salt-binding agents were introduced into clinical medicine in 1959 as a new weapon in the war against atherosclerosis [32]. Their development and introduction sprang directly from the realisation that bile salts are the major metabolic end-product of cholesterol and are essential for its absorption. It was hoped that accelerating the excretion of the end-product would increase cholesterol catabolism [650] and that this, together with reduced cholesterol absorption [592], would deplete the body stores of cholesterol. This hope has to a large extent been realised and this has stimulated the search for new and more active, safer and more palatable agents. Meanwhile other uses have been found for bile salt-binding agents, namely the treatment of pruritus caused by incomplete cholestasis and of diarrhoea caused by excessive passage of bile salts into the colon.

The essential features shared by all bile salt-binding agents are that they are high molecular weight compounds which are not absorbed to any significant extent. The way in which they bind bile salt molecules differs from one agent to another.

CHOLESTYRAMINE

This was the first bile salt-binding agent to be introduced [32] and it is by far the most widely used. It is a strongly basic (positively charged) anion exchange resin. Chemically it is a polystyrene polymer with a divinyl benzene cross linkage and quaternary ammonium groups in the chloride form. Its molecular weight is over a million [676]. It is believed to act by exchanging chloride ions for bile salt ions. Theoretically it is liable to bind other anions also, and it has been shown that the absorption of certain acidic drugs is depressed by the simultaneous administration of cholestyramine [208].

Surprisingly little *in vitro* work has been done with cholestyramine since the original demonstration by Tennent *et al.* [650] that it binds cholic acid in alcoholic solution. Whiteside *et al.* [698] showed that it binds about an equal weight of sodium cholate and most of the binding occurs within one minute. Taurocholate is bound somewhat more efficiently than glycocholate, but both tauro- and glycodeoxycholate are very well bound [261]. Steroid hormones [370] and porphyrins [623] are also bound.

Cholestyramine has been shown to sequestrate bile salts *in vivo* by several techniques. Firstly, it increases the faecal excretion of acidic steroids [91, 248, 448], while having little or no effect on neutral steroids (comprised mainly of cholesterol and its bacterial metabolites) [248, 448, 459]. Secondly, it accelerates the loss of labelled taurocholate and its metabolites from the bile [282, 354]. Thirdly, it increases the rate of decay of serum cholesterol specific activity which implies increased cholesterol turnover [248]; in the absence of increased excretion of neutral steroids this must indicate increased cholesterol catabolism. All these effects are identical to those resulting from ileal resection or bypass. Indeed the three- to eightfold elevation of faecal bile acids produced by cholestyramine [248, 448, 459] is the same as that produced by ileal dysfunction [186, 248, 709]. Similarly, in rats, cholestyramine treatment produces a marked rise in the liver activity of the rate-limiting reaction in bile acid synthesis, the 7α-hydroxylation of cholesterol [340].

That the upper small bowel is where cholestyramine binds bile salts is shown indirectly by the fact that this agent produces steatorrhoea if given to normal subjects in large doses (20-30 g daily) [161, 272, 713]. This steatorrhoea is mild to moderate and is relieved by administering an artificial detergent Tween 80 [161], or by feeding medium chain triglycerides [713] which are not dependent on micellar solubilisation. Since fat-soluble vitamins are very dependent on micellar solubilisation for their absorption, it is to be expected that this absorption will be interfered with by cholestyramine. Data on this point are very scanty. Certainly in 8-12 g doses cholestyramine lowers the peak rise in serum vitamin A following an oral load [24, 407]. Vitamin D and vitamin K absorption have been reduced in rats [660] and dogs [534] respectively. The occurrence of osteomalacia [284] and hypoprothrombinaemia [243] in occasional patients on cholestyramine suggests that fat-soluble vitamin absorption is impaired in man too, and emphasises the importance of giving supplements of these vitamins routinely to patients on this therapy.

The *therapeutic indications* for cholestyramine are now quite well defined. Of the hyperlipoproteinaemias only essential hypercholes-terolaemia (type II of Frederickson) responds well and here cholestyra-mine is probably the drug of choice [383]. It appears to be approximately as effective as ileal exclusion in lowering serum cholesterol levels when it is given in doses of 10-24 g/day, but both measures can fail when there is a marked rise in hepatic cholesterol synthesis [248, 459]. It also lowers the serum cholesterol of normal subjects [117, 713]. For some unexplained reason plasma triglycerides tend to rise [248]. It remains to be seen whether cholestyramine will alter the natural history of atherosclerosis as originally hoped.

The use of cholestyramine in the pruritus of incomplete cholestasis is also well established and it is particularly helpful in primary biliary cirrhosis [91, 128]. The dose can sometimes be reduced to 3.3 g/day [128]. Treated patients often show a fall in serum bilirubin and cholesterol and shrinkage of skin xanthomas, but the overall prognosis of the disease is not affected [128]. Relief of pruritus may take 5-10 days [88]. Obviously cholestyramine is of no value in complete biliary obstruction when there are no bile salts in the intestine for it to bind. However, it has been found helpful in children with intrahepatic bile duct atresia or 'ducto-penia' [577].

The use of cholestyramine in controlling the 'cholegenic' diarrhoea of ileal dysfunction was discussed on page 136.

The *effects of cholestyramine on bile itself* have recently attracted attention. The glycine/taurine conjugation ratio of bile salts (G/T ratio) is consistently increased, sometimes to 'pathological' levels [117, 282, 354]. This probably reflects the relative unavailability of taurine in the face of greatly increased demands for bile salt synthesis and hence for glycine and taurine side-chains, since the G/T ratio is also raised in ileal dysfunction and bile fistula (page 133). The tri-hydroxy/di-hydroxy ratio is also increased, so that glycocholate becomes the dominant bile salt [117, 282, 354, 675]. This is partly due to deoxycholate not being absorbed but there is also an unexplained reduction in chenodeoxy-cholate [117, 675]. The latter may be another hepatic response to enhanced bile salt synthesis, since a similar rise in the ratio of cholate to chenodeoxycholate occurs after the creation of a bile fistula [548]. The relative proportions of bile acids and phospholipid to cholesterol show inconstant changes in the short term [30, 675], but after six weeks they are said to be mildly to moderately decreased [117]. This is surprising since the bile salt pool appears to increase during cholestyramine therapy [354]. The effects of cholestyramine on the bile of animals are equally perplexing (see page 156).

LIGNIN

In 1967 Eastwood & Boyd showed that in the small intestine of rats a considerable amount of bile salt is associated with solid matter, especially if indigestible polysaccharide is added to the diet [164]. Eastwood went on to investigate the bile salt-binding properties of vegetable fibre *in vitro* [167]. The maize-barley residue left after manufacture of maltings for whisky ('dry grain') was shown to have significant bile acid-binding properties. Binding was greater with free than conjugated and with di-hydroxy than tri-hydroxy bile acids, and was increased by lowering the pH, which indicated non-polar or hydrophobic binding (in contrast to the ionic binding of cholestyramine). When the dry grain was treated to remove its various mainly polysaccharide components, it was found that only removal of lignin abolished its bile acid-binding properties. Lignin extracted from wood had these same properties, and they were enhanced by methylation of its phenolic hydroxyl groups (making it less polar) which again suggests hydrophobic bonding. Fibre from bran, fruit and vegetables had similar binding properties. It is noteworthy that binding was relatively slow compared with cholestyramine. After 5 min only 3 per cent of the binding had occurred, and 50 per cent by 30 min. Binding was not complete with taurocholate for 150 min.

These interesting studies established that lignin (which is not a polysaccharide but an amorphous phenylpropane polymer) has bile acid-binding properties *in vitro*, but these have not yet been demonstrated *in vivo*. In a straight weight-for-weight comparison in three normal subjects, lignin was found by Heaton *et al.* [282] to lack cholestyramine's readily demonstrated ability to remove radioactive taurocholate and its labelled metabolites from the enterohepatic circulation. Since these metabolites originate from free bile acids and are mainly conjugated with glycine, it was concluded that *in vivo* lignin has little or no ability to sequester the main circulating bile acids. If lignin binds conjugated bile salts it should interfere with lipid absorption. However, Barnard & Heaton [24] have found no consistent effect of lignin on the rise in serum vitamin A after an oral load, even when 12 g which is two to three times the suggested daily dose were mixed with the test meal. On the other hand, 12 g of cholestyramine (equivalent to a fairly small daily dose) always impaired vitamin A absorption, often to an impressive degree.

In spite of these negative results, claims have been made that lignin has therapeutic value in two situations where cholestyramine is effective. Eastwood has found lignin controls cholegenic diarrhoea in most patients with ileal resection [165, 166], though at the time of writing adequate documentation is still lacking. The author has compared it with cholestyramine in five patients and found it distinctly less effective [282]. A sixth patient found it more active than cholestyramine. Thiffault *et al.* [654] have given lignin to six patients with type II hyperlipidaemia and in all cases it either reduced serum cholesterol or maintained a reduction produced by cholestyramine. Remarkably, lignin was effective in the very small dose of 1.2 g daily. It is to be hoped that these important results will soon be confirmed.

If lignin is indeed therapeutically active, an explanation must be found for its apparent inactivity in the studies in normal subjects mentioned above. The following points seem relevant.

(1) Lignin binds rather slowly *in vitro*. If small intestinal transit is abnormally slow in type II hyperlipoproteinaemia, as postulated on page 171, then in this disease a longer time will be available for lignin to bind bile salts before they reach the ileal transport system. This could explain the effectiveness of lignin in type II hyperlipidaemia and its probable ineffectiveness in normocholesterolaemic subjects [163], as well as its lack of effect on circulating bile salts in normal subjects [282].

(2) Lignin should be particularly good at binding lithocholic acid, the least polar bile acid. Lithocholic acid may be involved in cholegenic diarrhoea, though this is unlikely in view of its insolubility. If absorbed, lithocholate can certainly cause hypercholesterolaemia in animals, probably by blocking cholesterol catabolism [328]. The studies on circulating bile salts mentioned above [282] would not have detected any effect of lignin on lithocholate.

(3) The one patient in whom lignin has been well documented as

controlling diarrhoea was a patient with massive resection of the distal small intestine [166]. In such patients the stool contains normal amounts of deoxycholate and little cholate, whereas with lesser resections the stool and bile tend to contain cholate and little deoxycholate (A. F. Hofmann, personal communication). It is to be expected that lignin will bind deoxycholate better than cholate, so its effects may only be striking with larger resections.

(4) Lignin may conceivably act by binding other as yet unidentified substances.

OTHER BILE SALT-BINDING AGENTS

Various cellulose and dextran anion exchangers bind bile salts *in vitro*. Of these, diethylaminoethyl (DEAE) cellulose, guanidoethyl cellulose and DEAE Sephadex have been shown to reduce experimental hypercholesterolaemia in cockerels [504]. In addition DEAE Sephadex reduced serum cholesterol in normocholesterolaemic dogs and increased faecal bile acid excretion [504]. Recently it has been reported that DEAE Sephadex is as effective as cholestyramine in lowering the serum cholesterol of elderly patients with type II hyperlipoproteinaemia, and that it is particularly effective when combined with clofibrate [325]. It is said to be more palatable than cholestyramine and virtually free of side effects [325] so it may well become a useful alternative drug.

Neomycin, and to a lesser extent kanamycin and paromomycin, precipitate bile salts *in vitro* [184], and especially dihydroxy bile salts [99]. Neomycin has definite hypocholesterolaemic properties. These may be attributed to increased bile acid excretion [542], but could be due in part to the production of a non-specific malabsorption syndrome [184] and to precipitation of mixed micelles [658].

Other agents which have been shown to interfere with bile salt absorption are colchicine [542], ferric salts [592] and certain alkaloids such as quinine and brucine [649]. However, these substances are absorbed and are too toxic for clinical use. Calcium carbonate may induce the precipitation of glycine conjugates [314], and there is a little evidence that pectin impairs bile salt absorption [390]. Benzmalecene is a drug which interferes with the active transport of bile salts [377].

The bulk-producing laxative psyllium hydrocolloid (Metamucil) increases bile salt excretion and lowers serum cholesterol [194], but this could be due to a physical action on the intestinal contents or transit rate rather than to chemical binding of bile salts. This agent has been shown to accelerate bile salt turnover and expand the bile salt pool size in rats [28]. Its action is probably analogous to that of dietary fibre.

16   Diet, Bile and Bile Salts

The motivation behind most investigations of the effect of different diets on bile and bile salts has been the belief that the high incidence of atherosclerosis and of gallstones in modern western society is dietary in origin and mediated through abnormal metabolism of cholesterol and of bile salts. Since the epidemiology of atherosclerosis and gallstones is so similar it is even possible that both diseases have a common dietary aetiology.

The main respects in which the Western diet has been alleged to be harmfully abnormal (apart from the use of chemical additives) are:

(1) It is too rich in cholesterol.
(2) It is too rich in fat, especially saturated fat.
(3) It is too highly processed.
(4) It contains too little vegetable fibre.
(5) It contains too much refined or highly available carbohydrate.

Each of these dietary factors will be considered in respect of their known or probable effects on bile salt metabolism and bile composition.

Since the intestinal lumen is the one place where bile salts and endogenous cholesterol meet the environment, in the form of the diet, it is important to consider especially carefully the effects of different diets on the recirculation of bile salts and on the absorption of cholesterol.

DIETARY CHOLESTEROL

In certain animals, such as dogs and rats, increasing the dietary intake of cholesterol results in increased bile acid production [149] and this seems to protect the animal from experimental atherosclerosis.

Most workers have failed to demonstrate any effect of dietary cholesterol on bile salt turnover in man, either by isotope turnover studies [287] or by sterol or isotope balance techniques [527, 702], but recently a 4 per cent cholesterol diet was said to nearly double faecal bile acids in young Indian girls [584].

As for the composition of the bile, again no consistent changes have been reported. In most of the healthy young volunteers studied by Dam et al. [118], there was actually a rise in the bile salt/cholesterol and lecithin/cholesterol ratios in duodenal aspirates after the subjects had eaten a diet containing 1-2 g of cholesterol for six weeks. The composition of the bile salt pool was not significantly altered. Studying a single patient, Sarles et al. [551] found no change in the lipid composition of hepatic bile when the diet was supplemented with 1.5 g of cholesterol daily. In contrast, other workers gave a patient 1 g of cholesterol daily for three months in addition to a formula diet and the bile became supersaturated with cholesterol [139]. In 11 subjects studied over three-week periods, adding 750 mg cholesterol daily to a formula diet caused a fall in bile acid secretion and a rise in cholesterol secretion, but also a rise in phospholipid secretion [139]. Thus the situation regarding the effects of dietary cholesterol in man remains confused. Studies using formula diets must be interpreted with caution since these diets of themselves alter bile salt metabolism (see below). With this in mind it is unlikely on present evidence that dietary cholesterol plays a part in the aetiology of gallstones.

It is not surprising if cholesterol feeding has little effect, since in man dietary cholesterol is poorly absorbed (probably because the absorptive mechanisms are already saturated with the normal load of endogenous cholesterol) [61].

In animals, added cholesterol is an integral part of certain atherogenic diets which also lead to the formation of cholesterol gallstones [496, 651]. However, an essential feature of these diets, as of most gallstone-producing diets [65], is that they are synthetic, rich in sugar or starch and lacking in fibre. In hamsters, adding cholesterol to such a synthetic diet actually reduces its lithogenicity [119].

AMOUNT OF FAT IN THE DIET

There is no convincing evidence that human bile salt turnover and metabolism are affected by the amount of fat in the diet. Ali et al. measured the faecal bile acids of three men on a totally fat-free diet [5]

and found them to be the same as on a diet rich in butter [6]. Similarly, Gordon *et al.* [288] found the faecal bile acids of seven subjects to be virtually identical on diets containing 8 g and 75 or 100 g of saturated fat. This is particularly noteworthy since faecal fat was higher on the high-fat diet. The amount of fibre in the diet may influence the response to different amounts of fat [10].

In rabbits, the change from a low-fat (normal) diet to a synthetic diet containing 26 per cent fat was associated with a fall in bile salt excretion [293]. This suggests that any effect of fat on bile salt turnover is small compared with that induced by a change to a synthetic diet (see below).

The concentrations of cholesterol and bile acids in human bile are not affected by the amount of fat in the diet, at least in short-term experiments [553]. Diets designed to induce gallstones in animals are generally low in fat content [177, 496] or even free of fat [113, 295]. It is unlikely therefore that high fat intake is the cause of human cholelithiasis.

In monkeys with controlled access to the common bile duct, the daily secretion of bile salts is lower on a low fat intake than on a high-fat diet, probably because there are fewer enterohepatic circulations [84]. It remains to be seen whether this is due to reduced gallbladder emptying.

In acute experiments, cholesterol absorption is increased by feeding fat [61, 665], presumably because the fat provides fatty acid and monoglyceride for the formation of mixed micelles. Also fatty acid is required for the esterification of cholesterol in the mucosa, prior to incorporation into chylomicrons [659].

TYPE OF FAT—SATURATED AND UNSATURATED

In an attempt to explain the hypocholesterolaemic action of polyunsaturated fat many workers have compared bile salt turnover on diets rich in saturated and polyunsaturated fat. The results have been conflicting and inconclusive.

Early studies in which faecal bile acids were found to be increased on unsaturated fat diets [10, 228, 229, 276] have been criticised [6, 246] in that the methods used (titrimetric, spectrophotometric) were too non-specific. Using the most refined techniques for estimating faecal bile acids, two groups of American workers have recently come

to opposite conclusions. Connor *et al.* [108] found that, after three weeks on a formula diet containing 40 per cent of calories as fat, faecal bile acids in six normal men averaged 271 mg daily when the fat was cocoa butter (saturated) and 426 mg when the fat was corn oil (unsaturated). This difference in bile acid excretion (together with an increase in neutral steroid excretion) was considered to be more than enough to explain the observed effect of corn oil on serum cholesterol. On the other hand, Grundy & Ahrens [245] found no change in bile acid excretion in eight of 11 patients with hyperlipoproteinaemia while their serum cholesterol was falling under the influence of unsaturated fat. On these and other grounds, they concluded that unsaturated fat acts by causing plasma cholesterol to be redistributed into tissue pools [245]. A similar conclusion was reached by Swedish workers after careful studies had failed to show any effect of different fats on faecal bile acids [125].

Equally inconclusive results have been obtained from investigations of bile salt turnover using isotopic techniques. Using the isotope derivative method (page 91) Avigan & Steinberg [18] found the average bile acid excretion of six hypercholesterolaemic subjects to be *lower*, but not significantly so, on unsaturated than on saturated fat. On the other hand, using the same method, Moore *et al.* [447] found faecal bile acids to be significantly higher on unsaturated fat in five normal young men, and Wood *et al.* [708] made the same observation in older subjects. Lindstedt and his colleagues hoped to solve the problem by measuring cholic acid turnover with the isotope dilution method. However, in extensive studies using solid and liquid diets in both normal subjects and hypercholesterolaemic patients, they were unable to correlate changes in serum cholesterol with changes in cholic acid turnover [289, 402]. Chenodeoxycholic acid turnover was not measured, but there was a slight tendency for the amount of this bile acid to decrease on unsaturated fat.

Animal studies such as those of Hellström *et al.* in rabbits [293] have added to the conviction [125] that bile acid excretion is not governed by the type of dietary fat. In rats, increased bile acid excretion has on occasions been noted with unsaturated fat [82], but this can be attributed to the fact that cholesterol was absorbed more efficiently when given together with unsaturated fat than when given with saturated fat [82, 659].

Investigations of the effect of different fats on the lipid composition

of bile have again yielded conflicting results. Watanabe *et al.* [686] claimed that feeding polyunsaturated fatty acids and pyridoxine to patients with T-tubes increased the lecithin content and therefore the cholesterol-holding power of the T-tube bile. Similarly, Redinger *et al.* [529] have reported that, in monkeys, feeding safflower oil doubles the bile salt pool size, enhances the secretion of phospholipid and increases the cholesterol-holding capacity of the bile. On the other hand, Sarles *et al.* [553] reported no change in the cholesterol or bile salt concentrations of T-tube bile in patients changing from saturated to unsaturated fat, while Dam *et al.* [114] found the lipid composition of duodenal aspirates from normal volunteers to be unaffected by three-week periods on butter-rich or linoleic acid-rich diets.

Two considerations throw doubt on the clinical significance of many studies with saturated and unsaturated fats. Firstly, the quantities of fat consumed by the volunteers (40-60 per cent of total calories) tend to be far higher than the normal dietary intake, which in any case involves a wide variety of different fats. Secondly, when liquid formula diets or other very refined diets are used a highly abnormal situation is produced. There is good evidence, reviewed below, that such refined diets of themselves have important effects on bile salt metabolism. It may also be questioned whether it was relevant to concentrate on diet fat in attempting to throw light on atherosclerosis and gallstones. The increase in fat consumption that has occurred in the U.S.A. during the period when these diseases have become so much more common has been slight, and largely confined to the very unsaturated fats which are believed to be preventive of these diseases [9].

These considerations, together with the confusing results of fat studies, suggest that the time has come to look for different dietary factors in trying to relate atherosclerosis and gallstones to altered bile salt metabolism.

SYNTHETIC AND FORMULA DIETS VERSUS 'NATURAL' DIETS

The consumption of highly processed and even synthetic foods is increasing in Western countries and in developing nations. It is desirable therefore to examine the effects of such diets on bile salt and cholesterol metabolism.

It was first noted by Portman *et al.* that rats eating a synthetic diet, which was nutritionally 'complete' and allowed normal growth, had a smaller pool size and lower excretion of bile salts than rats on a normal 'chow' diet [521, 524, 525]. The half-life of labelled cholic acid was prolonged from 2.0 to 3.2 days when the dietary carbohydrate was starch, and to 4.2 days when it was sucrose [525], indicating that bile salts were being absorbed abnormally efficiently. The small pool size and turnover rate implied decreased synthesis of bile salts. These findings were confirmed by other workers [256, 380]. Thus Gustafsson & Norman [256] found decreased bile acid excretion and prolonged cholate half-life in rats on a starch-based semi-synthetic diet. In rabbits too, the change from a normal pellet diet to a semi-synthetic diet is associated with a prolonged half-life and decreased excretion of bile acid [293].

In man there have been no direct comparisons of the effects of synthetic and 'natural' diets. However, Lindstedt *et al.* [402] noted that deoxycholate was absent from the bile in three out of five subjects taking a liquid formula diet, but in only one out of nine subjects on a solid diet. Three subjects were studied on transition from solid to liquid diets. In two the deoxycholate content of the bile fell, while in the third it was already absent. Since deoxycholate is produced in the colon, these data suggest that on a liquid formula diet there is reduced entry of bile salts into the colon. Clearly more studies are needed, but it is reasonable to suppose that reduced entry of bile salts into the colon may be associated with reduced bile salt excretion.

It is probable therefore that in man, as in animals, eating a synthetic diet diminishes bile salt excretion and so reduces cholesterol catabolism. In rats and hamsters on such a diet there is also increased liver synthesis of cholesterol [455, 295]. In several species, cholesterol levels in blood or bile can be made to rise markedly by feeding semi-synthetic diets [113, 521]. With the help of small additional dietary manipulations, actual cholelithiasis or atheroma can be induced. For example, hamsters can be made to form cholesterol gallstones by making their semi-synthetic diet fat-free [113, 295]; monkeys, which already show a marked rise in the bile cholesterol/phospholipid ratio on a basal semi-synthetic diet, can be made to develop cholelithiasis and atheroma when this diet is supplemented with butter and cholesterol [496]; dogs can be made to form gallstones by making the artificial diet low in protein and adding cholesterol [177]; and mice can be made to develop

cholelithiasis and atherosclerosis when the semi-synthetic diet is supplemented with cholesterol and cholic acid [651]. Conversely, adding 1 per cent cholesterol had a hypercholesterolaemic effect in rats only if the animals were fed a synthetic diet [533].

These various diets have two features in common. The first is a large proportion (50-72 per cent) of refined, or highly available carbohydrate, usually in the form of sucrose or glucose, sometimes refined starch. The second is the absence or virtual absence of plant fibre.

This suggests that synthetic diets induce the metabolic defects noted above, either through their lack of fibre or through their content of refined carbohydrate. There are grounds for incriminating both these dietary factors as capable of altering bile salt and cholesterol metabolism. These will now be discussed in turn.

PLANT FIBRE

All parts of plants contain fibre. Fibre consists of complex, mainly polysaccharide, polymers whose functions are to support, strengthen and protect the plant's structure. Cellulose is the main component but it is always accompanied by one or more of the following: pentosans or hemicelluloses, pectin and lignin. Nutritionists refer to cellulose and hemicelluloses as unavailable carbohydrates because in man they are not digested and absorbed, though they are to some extent metabolised by intestinal bacteria. Effects on bile salts and/or cholesterol metabolism have been recorded with crude fibre, cellulose, pectin and lignin. All four have hypocholesterolaemic activity, and very probably all four promote bile salt excretion and therefore cholesterol catabolism.

Adding pure cellulose to the diet as a 20 per cent supplement was shown by Portman & Murphy [525] largely to correct the depressed bile salt turnover of rats on a semi-synthetic high sucrose diet. This was due to a shortening of the prolonged cholic acid half-life. These findings were confirmed in germ-free rats by Gustafsson & Norman [256] (they found little effect of cellulose on conventional rats, possibly because the carbohydrate fed was not sucrose but starch which is less readily available though still refined). Similarly Sundaravalli et al. [632] found that in rats on a hypercholesterolaemic regime replacing cornstarch in the diet with cellulose to the 20 per cent level more than doubled the excretion of bile acids in the faeces. At the same time the usual rise in plasma and liver cholesterol was largely prevented. The same workers

have gone on to give 20 per cent cellulose (that is 100 g daily) to young girls on a hypercholesterolaemic regime, and have again shown increased bile acid excretion and prevention of hyperlipidaemia [584]. There can be no doubt therefore that cellulose does accelerate bile salt turnover when added to the diet in very large quantities, and presumably this explains its hypocholesterolaemic action.

Whole fibre probably has the same effect in man since Antonis & Bersohn [10] showed faecal bile acids to be 24-43 per cent higher on a low-fat diet containing about 15 g fibre than on a similar diet containing 4 g fibre. Much more work is needed along these lines. However, there is good evidence that plasma cholesterol is lower on a high fibre than a low fibre intake [666]. This statement applies to the geographical distribution of human plasma cholesterol levels as well as to the results of animal experiments.

Pectin has hypocholesterolaemic properties [356], and there is a little evidence that it increases bile acid excretion [390]. Lignin has been shown in a small trial to lower plasma cholesterol levels of patients with type II hyperlipoproteinaemia [654], but it has not yet been shown how it affects bile salt excretion.

The mode of action of fibre on bile salt turnover is uncertain. However, there is evidence from rat experiments that bile salts tend to be retained in the small bowel lumen when there is much cellulose in the diet [164]. This may be simply because the bowel contents are more voluminous, or because bile salts are trapped in the interstices of the polysaccharide mesh or gel. In either case absorption will be delayed or hindered. Since at the same time the transit rate through the intestine is likely to be more rapid, overall the reabsorption of bile salts will be reduced and their excretion increased. This simple physical-mechanical explanation is supported by two facts:

(1) All kinds of mucilaginous or gel-forming polysaccharides have hypocholesterolaemic properties [182]. One of them, psyllium hydrocolloid (Metamucil), which is widely used as a bulk-producing laxative, has in fact been shown to increase bile salt excretion in man [194], and to accelerate bile salt turnover and modestly increase bile salt pool size in rats [28].

(2) On diets of high fibre content there is reduced absorption of nutrients such as fat and nitrogen [616], which suggests that the effect of fibre is non-specific.

Chemical binding is another mechanism whereby fibre could increase bile salt excretion. *In vitro* it has been shown that whole fibre from cereal, vegetable and fruit sources has bile salt-binding properties, and that this capacity resides mainly in the lignin fraction [167]. Feeding purified lignin had no detectable effect on the rate of disappearance of circulating bile acids in three normal subjects [282]. However, this may merely mean that bile salts need to be trapped in a polysaccharide gel to allow time for the relatively slow binding action of lignin to be effective. Theoretically, cellulose which has ion-exchange properties, should bind bile salts. In rats on synthetic diets, adding 20 per cent pure cellulose to the diet did not increase the proportion of caecal and faecal bile salts bound to solid matter, even when this binding was initially low, as in germ-free rats [255]. Again, however, it is not safe to extrapolate from powdered cellulose (made from cotton) to cellulose in its natural state in food.

Bile acids vary in their tendency to be bound by fibre *in vitro,* the degree of binding being greatest with the least polar bile acids [167]. On this basis the circulating bile acid most affected by fibre should be lithocholic acid. This may be important in view of the ability of lithocholate to impair hepatic cholesterol metabolism (see also pages 124 and 159).

There is evidence in man [10] and rats [106] that cholesterol absorption is reduced by a high fibre intake, but this very important point does not seem to have been investigated by the best modern techniques. Theoretically an effect would be expected, since much if not most of the cholesterol in the small intestinal lumen is present in an undissolved state and after centrifugation is found in the sediment [418]. In this form it is presumably liable to be trapped by fibre and if it is carried to the ileum it will be irretrievably lost, since there are no more bile salt-fatty acid-monoglyceride micelles available to solubilise it. Any plant sterols (such as β-sitosterol) associated with the fibre will also tend to interfere with cholesterol absorption [245a].

The effects of dietary fibre on bile lipid ratios have not been reported at the time of writing. In view of all the above, there is clearly an urgent need for research on the effects of dietary fibre.

REFINED CARBOHYDRATE

To explain all the effects of synthetic diets on bile acid and cholesterol metabolism it is necessary to postulate an additional factor besides fibre lack, namely an effect on liver metabolism of the refined or rapidly available carbohydrate itself. (Rapidly available carbohydrate is the other side of the coin of fibre depletion, since the refining process by which it is obtained consists of treating the natural product in such a way as to separate the 'pure' carbohydrate-rich fraction from the fibre-rich fraction. Examples of carbohydrate refining are the manufacture of sucrose and of white flour [103].) The reasons for this are as follows:

(1) The deleterious effects of synthetic diets are not wholly reversed by supplementing the diet with fibre.

(2) The pathogenic effects of synthetic diets tend to be proportional to the degree of availability of their carbohydrate component.

(3) These effects are evident (in terms of cholesterol gallstone formation) in the dog [177], which being a carnivore does not normally ingest fibre at all. Therefore the cause of its gallstones cannot be fibre deficiency.

The first and second of these reasons require amplification.

(1) That the deleterious effects of synthetic diets are not wholly reversed by supplementing the diet with fibre is evident from the early experiments of Portman & Murphy [525]. In their rats eating a synthetic diet, the bile salt pool was much diminished, and it was not increased at all by feeding 20 per cent cellulose, even though the cholic acid half-life was shortened to subnormal levels. This suggests that cellulose failed to lift some factor suppressing bile salt synthesis. This suppression was in fact lifted by a 48-hour fast [524]. This makes it necessary to invoke a diet-related factor which directly inhibited hepatic synthesis. It may further be noted that, in another rat study, a semi-synthetic diet reduced the proportion of faecal bile salts bound to solid matter, but adding 20 per cent cellulose to the diet did not restore the binding to normal [255]. This raises the question of whether the factor inhibiting liver cholesterol catabolism on a synthetic diet is a faecal metabolite which is bound and excreted on a natural diet but is unbound and absorbed on a synthetic diet, even when cellulose is added. Lithocholate is an obvious candidate since it has a known ability to impair cholesterol catabolism.

(2) The effects of sugar-based diets tend to be greater than those of starch-based diets although in both cases there is total absence of fibre. In hamsters the tendency to form gallstones on a synthetic diet was

steadily reduced and eventually abolished as sucrose was replaced step-wise by rice-starch [113]. Bile composition showed parallel changes. In another investigation in hamsters hepatic cholesterol levels and synthesis rates were higher on sugar than on starch diets [295], while in rats a hypercholesterolaemic regime was more effective when the dietary carbohydrate was sucrose than when it was starch [523]. Sugars may be regarded as more rapidly available than starches since after sugar ingestion the plasma sugar and insulin rise higher, presumably because of quicker absorption [634]. The slower absorption of starch is probably the reason why the content of the hamster's intestine is much more voluminous on a starch diet than on a sugar diet [612]. Starch can be rendered soluble and therefore more quickly available by cooking, and it is of interest that in one investigation hamsters formed gallstones when their dietary carbohydrate was cooked starch, but not when it was raw starch [295].

Unfortunately there has been no work on the effects of sugar on cholesterol/bile acid metabolism since the old experimants of Wright & Whipple [711]. Using bile fistula dogs they showed that sugar induces a sharp drop in bile salt output and a lesser drop in cholesterol secretion. Recent work in monkeys [529] suggests that a high sugar intake reduces the size of the bile salt pool and the bile salt/cholesterol ratio. Sarles *et al.* [553] suggest that a high calorie intake can lead to an increased concentration of cholesterol in the bile. The mechanism of this change remains to be elucidated, but refined carbohydrate may well be a link in the chain.

The greater pathogenicity of refined sugar over refined starch may be linked with the fact that sugar production involves a greater degree of refining. Thus beet sugar is only 16 per cent of the whole beet while white flour is 70 per cent of the whole wheat grain.

The mode of action of refined carbohydrate on bile salt synthesis is quite unknown. However, it seems justifiable to speculate that rapid rises in blood sugar, and to counteract them in blood insulin, might lead to alterations in hepatic cholesterol metabolism [626, 627].

In summary there is much evidence that diets containing refined carbohydrate have adverse effects on cholesterol-bile acid metabolism. Some of these effects are attributable to fibre depletion, but some suggest a direct effect of rapidly available carbohydrate on hepatic metabolism. It seems best to consider the basic dietary abnormality as 'carbohydrate-refining'. This term encompasses all the effects discussed above and also accurately describes the manufacturing process which allows these effects to be produced.

OTHER DIETARY COMPONENTS AND BILE SALTS

Pyridoxine (vitamin B_6) deficiency has been shown to cause rats and monkeys, which normally conjugate only with taurine, to conjugate largely with glycine [522]. The relevance of this to human disease is uncertain.

Bibliography

1. Abaurre, R., Gordon, S. G., Mann, J. G. & Kern, F. (1969). Fasting bile salt pool size and composition after ileal resection. *Gastroenterology* **57**, 679-688.
2. Abell, L. L., Mosbach, E. H. & Kendall, F. E. (1956). Cholesterol metabolism in the dog. *J. biol. Chem.* **220**, 527-536.
3. Admirand, W. H. & Bauer, K. (1971). Phenobarbital (PB): an effective form of therapy in primary biliary cirrhosis. *J. clin. Invest.* **50**, 1A (abstract).
4. Admirand, W. H. & Small, D. M. (1968). The physicochemical basis of cholesterol gallstone formation in man. *J. clin. Invest.* **47**, 1043-1052.
5. Ali, S. S., Kuksis, A. & Beveridge, J. M. R. (1966a). Excretion of bile acids by three men on a fat-free diet. *Can. J. Biochem. Physiol.* **44**, 957-969.
6. Ali, S. S., Kuksis, A. & Beveridge, J. M. R. (1966b). Excretion of bile acids by three men on corn oil and butter fat diets. *Can. J. Biochem. Physiol.* **44**, 1377-1388.
7. Ament, M. E., Shimoda, S. S., Saunders, D. R. & Rubin, C. E. (1971). The pathogenesis of steatorrhea in stasis syndrome. *Gastroenterology* **60**, 637 (abstract).
7a. Anderson, K. E., Kok, E. & Javitt, N. B. (1972). Bile acid synthesis in man: metabolism of 7α-hydroxycholesterol-^{14}C and 26-hydroxycholesterol-^{3}H. *J. clin. Invest.* **51**, 112-117.
8. Andrews, E. & Aronsohn, H. G. (1936). Relative toxicity of different bile salts on the normal gall bladder. *Proc. Soc. exp. Biol. Med.* **34**, 765-767.
9. Antar, M. A., Ohlson, M. A. & Hodges, R. E. (1964). Changes in retail market food supplies in the United States in the last seventy years in relation to the incidence of coronary heart

disease, with special reference to dietary carbohydrates and essential fatty acids. *Am. J. clin. Nutr.* **14,** 169-178.

10. Antonis, A. & Bersohn, I. (1962). The influence of diet on fecal lipids in South African white and Bantu prisoners. *Am. J. clin. Nutr.* **11,** 142-155.

11. Arbuthnot, J. (1732). *An Essay Concerning the Nature of Aliments.* London: Tonson.

12. Arias, I. M. (1968). Formation of bile pigment. In *Handbook of Physiology,* Section 6: Alimentary Canal, Vol. V: Bile; digestion; ruminal physiology, ed. Code, C. F., pp. 2347-2374. Washington: American Physiological Society.

13. Aries, V. & Hill, M. J. (1970a). Degradation of steroids by intestinal bacteria. I. Deconjugation of bile salts. *Biochim. biophys. Acta* **202,** 526-534.

14. Aries, V. & Hill, M. J. (1970b). Degradation of steroids by intestinal bacteria. II. Enzymes catalysing the oxidoreduction of the 3α, 7α and 12α-hydroxyl groups in cholic acid, and the dehydroxylation of the 7-hydroxyl group. *Biochim. biophys. Acta* **202,** 535-543.

15. Arnesjö, B. (1971). The formation of lysolecithin in rat pancreas after experimentally induced bile salt pancreatitis. *Acta chir. scand.* **137,** 351-354.

16. Austad, W. I. (1970). Bile acid metabolism in hypercholesterolaemic subjects. *N.Z. med. J.* **71,** 237 (abstract).

17. Austad, W. I., Lack, L. & Tyor, M. P. (1967). Importance of bile acids and of an intact distal small intestine for fat absorption. *Gastroenterology* **52,** 638-646.

18. Avigan, J. & Steinberg, D. (1965). Steroid and bile acid excretion in man and the effect of dietary fat. *J. clin. Invest.* **44,** 1845-1856.

19. Badley, B. W. D., Murphy, G. M. & Bouchier, I. A. D. (1969). Intraluminal bile-salt deficiency in the pathogenesis of steatorrhoea. *Lancet* **2,** 400-402.

20. Badley, B. W. D., Murphy, G. M., Bouchier, I. A. D. & Sherlock, S. (1970). Diminished micellar phase lipid in patients with chronic non-alcoholic liver disease and steatorrhea. *Gastroenterology* **58,** 781-789.

21. Baker, R. D. & Searle, G. W. (1960). Bile salt absorption at various levels of rat small intestine. *Proc. Soc. exp. Biol. Med.* **105,** 521-523.

22. Balint, J. A., Beeler, D. A., Kyriakides, E. C. & Treble, D. H. (1971). The effect of bile salts upon lecithin synthesis. *J. Lab. clin. Med.* 77, 122-133.

23. Baraona, E., Palma, R., Navia, E., Salinas, A., Orrego, H. & Espinoza, J. (1968). The role of unconjugated bile salts in the malabsorption of glucose and tyrosine by everted sacs of jejunum of rats with the 'blind-loop syndrome'. *Acta physiol. latinoam.* 18, 291-297.

24. Barnard, D. & Heaton, K. W. (1971). Unpublished observations.

25. Barry, E. (1759). *A Treatise on the Three Different Digestions, and Discharges of the Human Body.* London: A. Miller.

26. Beaumont, W. (1838). *Experiments and Observations on the Gastric Juice, and the Physiology of Digestion.* Edinburgh: MacLachlan & Stewart.

27. Beck, I. T., Sum, P. & Bencosme, S. A. (1969). The study of the pathogenesis of bile induced acute pancreatitis in the dog. Experiments with detergent. *Gastroenterology* 56, 1247 (abstract).

28. Beher, W. T. & Casazza, K. K. (1971). Effects of psyllium hydrocolloid on bile acid metabolism in normal and hypophysectomised rats. *Proc. Soc. exp. Biol. Med.* 136, 253-256.

29. Beher, W. T., Filus, A. M., Rao, B. & Beher, M. E. (1969). A comparative study of bile acid metabolism in the rat, mouse, hamster and gerbil. *Proc. Soc. exp. Biol. Med.* 130, 1067-1074.

30. Beher, W. T., Schuman, B. M., Block, M. A. & Casazza, K. K. (1971). The effect of psyllium hydrocolloid and cholestyramine (Cuemid) on hepatic bile lipid ratios in man *Gastroenterology* 60, 191 (abstract).

30a. Bell, C. C., McCormick, W. C., Gregory, D. H., Law, D. H., Vlahcevic, Z. R. & Swell, L. (1972). Relationship of bile acid pool size to the formation of lithogenous bile in male Indians of the Southwest. *Surgery Gynec. Obstet.* 134, 473-478.

31. Bell, C. C., Vlahcevic, Z. R. & Swell, L. (1971). Alterations in the lipids of human hepatic bile after the oral administration of bile salts. *Surgery Gynec. Obstet.* 132, 36-42.

32. Bergen, S. S., van Itallie, T. B., Tennent, D. M. & Sebrell, W. (1959). Effect of an anion exchange resin on serum cholesterol in man. *Circulation* 20, 981 (abstract).

33. Bergman, F. & van der Linden, W. (1967). Diet-induced cholesterol gallstones in hamsters: prevention and dissolution by cholestyramine. *Gastroenterology* 53, 418-421.

34. Bergman, F. & van der Linden, W. (1968). Effect of cholestyramine on cholesterol gallstones in mice. *Acta chir. scand.* **134**, 287-291.

35. Bergman, F., van der Linden, W. & Sjövall, J. (1968). Biliary bile acids and hepatic ultra-structure in hamsters fed gallstone-inducing and -dissolving diets. *Acta physiol. scand.* **74**, 480-491.

36. Bergström, S. & Danielsson, H. (1958). On the regulation of bile acid formation in the rat liver. *Acta physiol. scand.* **43**, 1-7.

37. Bergström, S. & Danielsson, H. (1968). Formation and metabolism of bile acids. In *Handbook of Physiology,* Section 6: Alimentary Canal, Vol. 5: Bile; Digestion; Ruminal Physiology, ed. Code, C. F., pp. 2391-2407. Washington: American Physiological Society.

38. Bergström, S., Danielsson, H. & Samuelsson, B. (1960). Formation and metabolism of bile acids. In *Lipide Metabolism,* ed. Bloch, K., pp. 291-336. New York: Wiley.

39. Bergström, S. & Norman, A. (1953). Metabolic products of cholesterol in bile and feces of rat. *Proc. Soc. exp. Biol. Med.* **83**, 71-74.

40. Bergström, S., Rottenberg, M. & Voltz, J. (1953). The preparation of some carboxy labelled bile acids. *Acta chem. scand.* **7**, 481-484.

41. Berman, A. L., Snapp, E., Ivy, A. C. & Atkinson, A. J. (1941). On the regulation or homeostasis of the cholic acid output in biliary-duodenal fistula dogs. *Am. J. Physiol.* **131**, 776-782.

42. Bernard, C. (1856). Cited by Sobotka (1937).

43. Berthelot, P., Erlinger, S., Dhumeaux, D. & Preaux, A. M. (1970). Mechanism of phenobarbital-induced hypercholeresis in the rat. *Am. J. Physiol.* **219**, 809-813.

44. Berzelius (1809). Cited by Sobotka (1938).

45. Bidder, F. & Schmidt, C. (1852). *Die Verdauungssaefte und der Stoffwechsel.* Mitau und Leipzig: Reyher.

46. Biss, K., Ho, K.-J., Mikkelson, B., Lewis, L. & Taylor, C. B. (1971). Some unique biologic characteristics of the Masai of East Africa. *New Engl. J. Med.* **284**, 694-699.

47. Black, R. B., Hole, D. & Rhodes, J. (1971). Bile damage to the gastric mucosal barrier: the influence of pH and bile acid concentration. *Gastroenterology* **61**, 178-184.

48. Black, R. B., Roberts, G. & Rhodes, J. (1971). The effect of healing on bile reflux in gastric ulcer. *Gut* **12**, 552-558.

49. Bloch, K., Berg, B. N. & Rittenberg, D. (1943). The biological conversion of cholesterol to cholic acid. *J. biol. Chem.* **149**, 511-517.

50. Blomstrand, R., Carlberger, G. & Forsgren, L. (1969). Intestinal absorption and metabolism of ^{14}C-labelled fatty acids in the absence of bile in man. *Acta chir. scand.* **135**, 329-339.

51. Blum, M. & Spritz, N. (1966). The metabolism of intravenously injected isotopic cholic acid in Laennec's cirrhosis. *J. clin. Invest.* **45**, 187-193.

52. Booth, C. C., Alldis, D. & Read, A. E. (1961). Studies on the site of fat absorption. 2. Fat balances after resection of varying amounts of the small intestine in man. *Gut* 168-174.

53. Booth, C. C., MacIntyre, I. & Mollin, D. L. (1964). Nutritional problems associated with extensive lesions of distal small intestine in man. *Q. Jl Med.* **33**, 401-420.

54. Borgström, B. (1952). On the action of pancreatic lipase on triglycerides *in vivo* and *in vitro*. *Acta physiol. scand.* **25**, 328-347.

55. Borgström, B. (1954). Effect of tauro-cholic acid on the pH/activity curve of rat pancreatic lipase. *Biochim. biophys. Acta* **13**, 149-150.

56. Borgström, B. (1960). Studies on intestinal cholesterol absorption in the human. *J. clin. Invest.* **39**, 809-815.

57. Borgström, B. (1962). Digestion and absorption of fat. *Gastroenterology* **43**, 216-219.

58. Borgström, B. (1967). Partition of lipids between emulsified oil and micellar phases of glyceride-bile salt dispersions. *J. Lipid Res.* **8**, 598-608.

59. Borgström, B., Dahlqvist, A., Lundh, G. & Sjövall, J. (1957). Studies of intestinal digestion and absorption in the human. *J. clin. Invest.* **36**, 1521-1536.

60. Borgström, B., Lundh, G. & Hofmann, A. (1963). The site of absorption of conjugated bile salts in man. *Gastroenterology* **45**, 229-238.

61. Borgström, B., Radner, S. & Werner, B. (1970). Lymphatic transport of cholesterol in the human being. Effect of dietary cholesterol. *Scand. J. clin. Lab. Invest.* **26**, 227-235.

62. Bouchier, I. A. D. (1968). Gallstone formation and properties of bile. *Brit. J. Hosp. Med.* **1**, 33-39.

63. Bouchier, I. A. D. (1969). Postmortem study of the frequency of gallstones in patients with cirrhosis of the liver. *Gut* **10**, 705-710.

64. Bouchier, I. A. D. (1971a). Gallstone formation. *Lancet* **1**, 711-715.

65. Bouchier, I. A. D. (1971b). Experimental cholelithiasis. In *The Scientific Basis of Medicine Annual Reviews 1971*, ed. Gilliland, I. & Francis, J. pp. 232-243. London: Athlone Press.

66. Bouchier, I. A. D. (1971c). Personal communication.

67. Bouchier, I. A. D. & Cooperband, S. R. (1967). Isolation and characterisation of a macromolecular aggregate associated with bilirubin. *Clin. chim. Acta* **15**, 291-302.

68. Boyer, J. L. & Klatskin, G. (1970). Canalicular bile flow and bile secretory pressure. Evidence for a non-bile salt dependent fraction in the isolated perfused rat liver. *Gastroenterology* **59**, 853-859.

69. Bray, G. A. & Gallagher, T. F. (1968). Suppression of appetite by bile acids. *Lancet* **1**, 1066-1067.

70. Bremer, J. (1955). The conjugation of glycine with cholic acid and benzoic acid in rat liver homogenate. *Acta chem. scand.* **9**, 268-271.

71. Brooks, F. P. (1969). The secretion of bile. *Am. J. dig. Dis.* **14**, 343-349.

72. Brooks, F. P. (1970). *Control of Gastrointestinal Function.* London: MacMillan.

72a. Brunner, H., Hofmann, A. F. & Summerskill, W. H. J. (1972). Daily secretion of bile acids and cholesterol measured in health. *Gastroenterology* **62**, 188 (abstract).

73. Bruusgaard, A. (1970). Quantitative determination of the major 3-hydroxy bile acids in biological material after thin-layer chromatographic separation. *Clin. Chim. Acta* **28**, 495-504.

74. Bruusgaard, A. & Thaysen, E. H. (1970). Increased ratio of glycine/taurine conjugated bile acids in the early diagnosis of terminal ileopathy. Preliminary report. *Acta med. scand.* **188**, 547-548.

75. Buchwald, H. (1965). The effect of ileal bypass on atherosclerosis and hypercholesterolemia in the rabbit. *Surgery, St. Louis* **58**, 22-35.

76. Buchwald, H. & Varco, R. L. (1966). Ileal bypass in patients with hypercholesterolemia and atherosclerosis. *J. Am. med. Ass.* **196**, 627-630.

77. Budd, G. (1845). *On Diseases of the Liver.* London: Churchill.

78. Burke, C. W., Lewis, B., Panveliwalla, D. & Tabaqchali, S. (1971). The binding of cholic acid and its taurine conjugate to serum proteins. *Clin. chim. Acta* **32**, 207-214.

79. Burkitt, D. P. (1971). Epidemiology of cancer of the colon and rectum. *Cancer* **28**, 3-13.

81. Burnett, W. (1965). The pathogenesis of gallstones. In *The Biliary System,* ed. Taylor, W., pp. 601-618. Oxford: Blackwell.

82. Byers, S. O. & Friedman, M. (1958). Bile acid metabolism, dietary fats and plasma cholesterol levels. *Proc. Soc. exp. Biol. Med.* **98**, 523-526.

83. Caldwell, F. T. & Levitsky, K. (1967). The gallbladder and gallstone formation. *Ann. Surg.* **166**, 753-758.

84. Campbell, C. B., Spencer, J. & Dowling, R. H. (1969). Bile salt secretion and pool size in Rhesus monkeys with controlled interruption of the enterohepatic circulation. *Gut* **10**, 1050 (abstract).

85. Cardis, D. T., Roberts, M. & Smith, G. (1968). The effect of small bowel resection on gastric acid secretion in the rat. *Br. J. Surg.* **55**, 392 (abstract).

86. Carey, J. B. (1958). The serum trihydroxy-dihydroxy bile acid ratio in liver and biliary tract disease. *J. clin. Invest.* **37**, 1494-1503.

87. Carey, J. B. (1960). Lowering of serum bile acid concentrations and relief of pruritus in jaundiced patients fed a bile acid sequestering resin. *J. Lab. clin. Med.* **56**, 797-798 (abstract).

88. Carey, J. B. (1970). Bile salts and hepatobiliary disease. In *Diseases of the Liver,* ed. Schiff, L., 3rd edn, pp. 103-146. Philadelphia: Lippincott.

89. Carey, J. B. & Hanson, R. F. (1969). 3 alpha, 7 alpha, dihydroxy-coprostanic acid in human bile. In *Bile Salt Metabolism,* ed. Schiff, L., Carey, J. B. & Dietschy, J. M., pp. 5-12. Springfield: Thomas.

90. Carey, J. B. & Haslewood, G. A. D. (1963). Crystallisation of tri-hydroxy coprostanic acid from human bile. *J. biol. Chem.* **238**, PC 855-856.

91. Carey, J. B. & Williams, G. (1961). Relief of the pruritus of jaundice with a bile-acid sequestering resin. *J. Am. med. Ass.* **176**, 432-435.

92. Carey, J. B. & Williams, G. (1963). Metabolism of lithocholic acid in bile fistula patients. *J. clin. Invest.* **42**, 450-455.

93. Carey, J. B. & Williams, G. (1965). Lithocholic acid in human-blood serum. *Science* **150**, 620-622.

94. Carey, J. B. & Williams, G. (1969). Maximum primary bile salt synthesis rates in man. *Gastroenterology* **56**, A121 (abstract).

95. Carey, J. B., Wilson, I. D., Zaki, F. G. & Hanson, R. F. (1966). The metabolism of bile acids with special reference to liver injury. *Medicine, Baltimore* **45**, 461-470.

96. Carey, M. C. & Small, D. M. (1969). Micellar properties of dihydroxy and trihydroxy bile salts: Effects of counterion and temperature. *J. Colloid Interface Sci.* **31**, 382-396.

97. Carey, M. C. & Small, D. M. (1970). The characteristics of mixed micellar solutions with particular reference to bile. *Am. J. Med.* **49**, 590-608.

98. Cassells, J. S., Banwell, J. G., Gorbach, S. L., Mitra, R. & Guha Mazumder, D. N. (1970). Tropical sprue and malnutrition in West Bengal. IV. Bile salt deconjugation in tropical sprue. *Am. J. Clin. Nutr.* **23**, 1579-1581.

99. Cayen, M. N. (1970). Agents affecting lipid metabolism. XXXVIII. Effect of neomycin on cholesterol biosynthesis and bile acid precipitation. *Am. J. clin. Nutr.* **23**, 1234-1240.

100. Cesano, L. & Dawson, A. M. (1966). Absorption of ^{14}C triolein in the bile fistula rat. *Proc. Soc. exp. Biol. Med.* **122**, 96-99.

101. Cheney, F. E., Burke, V., Clark, M. L. & Senior, J. R. (1970). Intestinal fatty acid absorption and esterification from luminal micellar solutions containing deoxycholic acid. *Proc. Soc. exp. Biol. Med.* **133**, 212-215.

102. Clark, M. L., Lanz, H. C. & Senior, J. R. (1969). Bile salt regulation of fatty acid absorption and esterification in rat everted jejunal sacs *in vitro* and into thoracic duct lymph *in vivo*. *J. clin. Invest.* **48**, 1587-1599.

103. Cleave, T. L., Campbell, G. D. & Painter, N. S. (1969). *Diabetes, Coronary Thrombosis and the Saccharine Disease.* 2nd edn. Bristol: Wright.

104. Coe, T. (1757). *A Treatise on Biliary Concretions; Or, Stones in the Gall-Bladder and Ducts.* London: Wilson & Durham.

105. Cohen, S., Kaplan, M., Gottlieb, L. & Patterson, J. (1971). Liver disease and gallstones in regional enteritis. *Gastroenterology* **60**, 237-245.

106. Coleman, D. L. & Baumann, C. A. (1959). Intestinal sterols. III. Effects of age, sex and diet. *Archs Biochem. Biophys.* **66**, 226-233.

107. Columbus, Realdus (1572). *De Re Anatomica.* Paris: Wechelum.

108. Connor, W. E., Witiak, D. T., Stone, D. B. & Armstrong, M. L. (1969). Cholesterol balance and fecal neutral steroid and bile acid excretion in normal men fed dietary fats of different fatty acid composition. *J. clin. Invest.* **48**, 1363-1375.

109. Cooper, R. A. & Jandl, J. H. (1968). Bile salts and cholesterol in the pathogenesis of target cells in obstructive jaundice. *J. clin. Invest.* 47, 809-822.

110. Creutzfeldt, W. & Schmidt, H. (1970). Aetiology and pathogenesis of pancreatitis (current concepts). *Scand. J. Gastroent. Suppl.* 6, 47-62.

111. Cronholm, T., Norman, A. & Sjövall, J. (1970). Bile acids and steroid sulphates in serum of patients with infectious hepatitis. *Scand. J. Gastroent.* 5, 297-303.

112. Cronholm, T. & Sjövall, J. (1967). Bile acids in portal blood of rats fed different diets and cholestyramine. *Eur. J. Biochem.* 2, 375-383.

113. Dam, H. (1964). Nutritional factors in gallstone formation. In *Proceedings of the Sixth International Congress of Nutrition, Edinburgh 1963,* pp. 6-23. Edinburgh: Livingstone.

114. Dam, H., Kruse, I., Jensen, M. K. & Kallehauge, H. E. (1967). Studies on human bile. II. Influence of two different fats on the composition of human bile. *Scand. J. clin. Lab. Invest.* 19, 367-378.

115. Dam, H., Kruse, I., Kallehauge, H. E., Hartkopp, O. E. & Jensen, M. K. (1966). Studies on human bile. I. Composition of bladder bile from cholelithiasis patients and surgical patients with normal bile compared with data for bladder bile of hamsters on different diets. *Scand. J. clin. Lab. Invest.* 18, 385-404.

116. Dam, H., Kruse, I., Prange, I., Kallehauge, H. E., Fenger, H. J. & Jensen, M. K. (1971). Studies on human bile. III. Composition of duodenal bile from healthy young volunteers compared with composition of bladder bile from surgical patients with and without uncomplicated gallstone disease. *Z. Ernährungsw.* 10, 160-177.

117. Dam, H., Prange, I., Jensen, M. K., Kallehauge, H. E. & Fenger, H. J. (1971a). Studies on human bile. V. Influence of cholestyramine treatment on the composition of bile in healthy subjects. *Z. Ernährungsw.* 10, 188-197.

118. Dam, H., Prange, I., Jensen, M. K., Kallehauge, H. E. & Fenger, H. J. (1971b). Studies on human bile. IV. Influence of ingestion of cholesterol in the form of eggs on the composition of bile in healthy subjects. *Z. Ernährungsw.* 10, 178-187.

119. Dam, H., Prange, I. & Sondergaard, E. (1968). Alimentary production of gallstones in hamsters. 20. Influence of dietary cholesterol on gallstone formation. *Z. Ernährungsw.* 9, 43-49.

120. Danielsson, H. (1963). Present status of research on catabolism and excretion of cholesterol. *Adv. Lipid Res.* 1, 335-385.

121. Danielsson, H. (1969). Mechanisms of bile acid formation. In *Bile Salt Metabolism,* ed. Schiff, L., Carey, J. B. & Dietschy, J. M., pp. 91-102. Springfield: Thomas.

122. Danielsson, H. (1970). Paper given to the International Bile Salt Meeting, Freiburg, 5 October, 1970.

123. Danielsson, H., Einarsson, K. & Johansson, G. (1967). Effect of biliary drainage on individual reactions in the conversion of cholesterol to taurocholic acid. *Eur. J. Biochem.* 2, 44-49.

124. Danielsson, H., Eneroth, P., Hellström, K., Lindstedt, S. & Sjövall, J. (1963). On the turnover and excretory products of cholic and chenodeoxycholic acid in man. *J. biol. Chem.* 238, 2299-2304.

125. Danielsson, H. & Tchen, T. T. (1968). Steroid metabolism. In *Metabolic Pathways,* ed. Greenberg, D. M., Vol. 11: Lipids, steroids and carotenoids, 3rd edn., pp. 117-168. New York: Academic Press.

126. Danzinger, R. G., Hofmann, A. F., Schoenfield, L. J., Berngruber, O. W., Szczepanik, P. A. & Klein, P. D. (1971). Measurement of bile acid kinetics in man using stable isotopes: application to cholelithiasis. *Gastroenterology* 60, 192 (abstract).

127. Danzinger, R. G., Hofmann, A. F., Schoenfield, L. J. & Thistle, J. L. (1972). Dissolution of cholesterol gallstones by chenodeoxycholic acid. *New Engl. J. Med.* 286, 1-8.

128. Datta, D. V. & Sherlock, S. (1966). Cholestyramine for long term relief of the pruritus complicating intrahepatic cholestasis. *Gastroenterology* 50, 323-332.

129. Davenport, H. W. (1966). *Physiology of the digestive tract.* 2nd edn. Chicago: Year Book Medical Publishers.

130. Davenport, H. W. (1967). Absorption of taurocholate-24-C^{14} through the canine gastric mucosa. *Proc. Soc. exp. Biol. Med.* 125, 670-673.

131. Davenport, H. W. (1968). Destruction of the gastric mucosal barrier by detergents and urea. *Gastroenterology* 54, 175-181.

132. Davenport, H. W. (1970). Effect of lysolecithin, digitonin and phospholipase A upon the dog's gastric mucosal barrier. *Gastroenterology* 59, 505-509.

133. Davidson, S. & Passmore, R. (1969). *Human Nutrition and Dietetics,* 4th edn. Edinburgh: Livingstone.

134. Dawson, A. M. (1967). Bile salts and fat absorption. *Gut* 8, 1-3.

135. Dawson, A. M. & Isselbacher, K. J. (1960). Studies on lipid metabolism in the small intestine with observations on the role of bile salts. *J. clin. Invest.* **39**, 730-740.

136. Dawson, A. M. & Saunders, D. R. (1965). Effect of bile salts on the pathway of fat absorption in the rat. In *The Biliary System,* ed. Taylor, W., pp. 183-187. Oxford: Blackwell.

137. Dean, P. D. G. & Whitehouse, M. W. (1967). Inhibition of hepatic sterol oxidation by cholanic (bile) acids and their conjugates. *Biochim. biophys. Acta* **137**, 328-334.

138. Demarçay, H. (1838). Cited by Strecker (1848).

139. DenBesten, L. & Connor, W. E. (1971). Effect of dietary cholesterol on bile composition in man. *Gastroenterology* **60**, 654 (abstract).

140. Denk, H., Greim, H. & Hutterer, F. (1971). Detergent action of bile acids on hepatocellular microsomes, and its role in cholestasis. *Gastroenterology* **60**, 187 (abstract).

141. Desnuelle, P. (1961). Pancreatic lipase. *Adv. Enzymol.* **23**, 129-161.

142. Diemerbroek, I. (1683). *Anatome Corporis Humani.* Leiden: Huguetan.

143. Dietschy, J. M. (1966). Recent developments in solute and water transport across the gall-bladder epithelium. *Gastroenterology* **50**, 692-707.

144. Dietschy, J. M. (1967). Effects of bile salts on intermediate metabolism of the intestinal mucosa. *Fedn Proc.* **26**, 1589-1598.

145. Dietschy, J. M. (1968a). Mechanisms for the intestinal absorption of bile acids. *J. Lipid. Res.* **9**, 297-309.

146. Dietschy, J. M. (1968b). The role of bile salts in controlling the rate of intestinal cholesterogenesis. *J. clin. Invest.* **47**, 286-300.

147. Dietschy, J. M. & Gamel, W. G. (1971). Cholesterol synthesis in the intestine of man: regional differences and control mechanisms. *J. clin. Invest.* **50**, 872-880.

148. Dietschy, J. M., Salomon, H. S. & Siperstein, M. D. (1966). Bile acid metabolism. I. Studies on the mechanisms of intestinal transport. *J. clin. Invest.* **45**, 832-846.

149. Dietschy, J. M. & Wilson, J. D. (1970). Regulation of cholesterol metabolism. *New Engl. J. Med.* **282**, 1128-1138, 1179-1183, 1241-1249.

150. DiMagno, E. F., Go, V. L. W. & Summerskill, W. H. J. (1969). Pancreozymin secretion is impaired in sprue. *Gastroenterology* **56**, 1149 (abstract).

151. Donaldson, R. M. (1965). Studies on the pathogenesis of steatorrhea in the blind loop syndrome. *J. clin. Invest.* **44,** 1815-1825.

152. Donaldson, R. M. (1970). Small bowel bacterial overgrowth. *Adv. internal Med.* **16,** 191-212.

153. Dowling, R. H. (1970). Small bowel resection and bypass—recent developments and effects. In *Modern Trends in Gastroenterology—4,* ed. Card, W. I. & Creamer, B., pp. 73-104. London: Butterworths.

154. Dowling, R. H., Mack, E. & Small, D. M. (1970). Effects of controlled interruption of the enterohepatic circulation of bile salts by biliary diversion and by ileal resection on bile salt secretion, synthesis and pool size in the Rhesus monkey. *J. clin. Invest.* **49,** 232-242.

155. Dowling, R. H., Mack, E. & Small, D. M. (1971). Biliary lipid secretion and bile composition after acute and chronic interruption of the enterohepatic circulation in the Rhesus monkey. IV. Primate biliary physiology. *J. clin. Invest.* **50,** 1917-1926.

155a. Dowling, R. H., Rose, G. A. & Sutor, D. J. (1971). Hyperoxaluria and renal calculi in ileal disease. *Lancet* **1,** 1103-1106.

156. Dowling, R. H. & Small, D. M. (1968). The effect of pH on the solubility of varying mixtures of free and conjugated bile salts in solution. *Gastroenterology* **54,** 1291 (abstract).

157. Dowse, C. M., Saunders, J. A. & Schofield, B. (1956). The composition of lipid from jejunal contents of the dog after a fatty meal. *J. Physiol.* **134,** 515-526.

158. Drasar, B. S., Hill, M. J. & Shiner, M. (1966). The deconjugation of bile salts by human intestinal bacteria. *Lancet* **1,** 1237-1238.

159. Drasar, B. S. & Shiner, M. (1969). Studies on the intestinal flora. Part II. Bacterial flora of the small intestine in patients with gastro-intestinal disorders. *Gut* **10,** 812-819.

160. Dreher, K. D., Schulman, J. H. & Hofmann, A. F. (1967). Surface chemistry of the monoglyceride-bile salt system: its relationship to the function of bile salts in fat absorption. *J. Colloid Interface Sci.* **25,** 71-83.

161. DuBois, J. J., Holt, P. R., Kuron, G. W., Hashim, S. A. & van Itallie, T. B. (1964). Effect of Tween 80 on cholestyramine-induced malabsorption. *Proc. Soc. exp. Biol. Med.* **117,** 226-229.

162. Earnest, D. E. & Admirand, W. H. (1971). The effects of individual bile salts in cholesterol solubilisation and gallstone dissolution. *Gastroenterology* **60**, 772 (abstract).

163. Eastwood, M. (1969). Dietary fibre and serum lipids. *Lancet* **2**, 1222-1224.

164. Eastwood, M. A. & Boyd, G. S. (1967). The distribution of bile salts along the small intestine of rats. *Biochim. biophys. Acta* **137**, 393-396.

165. Eastwood, M. A. & Eriksson, S. (1970). The use of lignin in controlling diarrhoea due to ileal dysfunction. *Gut* **11**, 370 (abstract).

166. Eastwood, M. A. & Girdwood, R. H. (1968). Lignin: a bile-salt sequestrating agent. *Lancet* **2**, 1170-1171.

167. Eastwood, M. A. & Hamilton, D. (1968). Studies on the adsorption of bile salts to non-absorbed components of diet. *Biochim. biophys. Acta* **152**, 165-173.

168. Eguchi, T. (1965). Studies on pathogenesis of cholesterol gallstones, especially with respect to behaviour of cholesterol metabolism. *Arch. jap. Chir.* **34**, 1181-1195.

169. Einarsson, K. & Johansson, G. (1968). Effect of phenobarbital on the conversion of cholesterol to taurocholic acid. *Eur. J. Biochem.* **6**, 293-298.

170. Ekdahl, P.-H. (1958). On the conjugation and formation of bile acids in the human liver. VI. On the conjugation of cholic acid-24^{14}C in human liver homogenates in various diseases with special reference to patients with jaundice. *Acta chir. scand.* **115**, 208-226.

171. Ekdahl, P.-H. & Gloor, U. (1958). On the conjugation and formation of bile acids in the human liver. II. On the conjugation of cholic acid (-24^{14}C) in human liver homogenates. *Acta chir. scand.* **114**, 453-460.

172. Ekdahl, P.-H. & Sjövall, J. (1958). On the conjugation and formation of bile acids in the human liver. I. On the excretion of bile acids by patients with postoperative choledochostomy drainage. *Acta chir. scand.* **114**, 439-452.

172a. Elliott, W. H. & Hyde, P. M. (1971). Metabolic pathways of bile acid synthesis. *Am. J. Med.* **51**, 568-579.

173. Encrantz, J.-C. & Sjövall, J. (1959). On the bile acids in duodenal contents of infants and children. *Clin. chim. Acta* **4**, 793-799.

174. Eneroth, P. (1963). Thin-layer chromatography of bile acids. *J. Lipid Res.* **4**, 11-16.

175. Eneroth, P. (1969). Thin-layer chromatography of bile alcohols and bile acids. In *Lipid Chromatographic Analysis,* ed. Marinetti, G. V., Vol. 2, pp. 149-186. New York: Dekker.

176. Eneroth, P., Gordon, B., Ryhage, R. & Sjövall, J. (1966). Identification of mono- and dihydroxy bile acids in human feces by gas-liquid chromatography and mass spectrometry. *J. Lipid Res.* 7, 511-523.

177. Englert, E., Harman, C. G. & Wales, E. E. (1969). Gallstones induced by normal foodstuffs in dogs. *Nature, Lond.* 224, 280-281.

178. Eriksson, S. (1957a). Biliary excretion of bile acids and cholesterol in bile fistula rats. *Proc. Soc. exp. Biol. Med.* 94, 578-582.

179. Eriksson, S. (1957b). Influence of thyroid activity on excretion of bile acids and cholesterol in the rat. *Proc. Soc. exp. Biol. Med.* 94, 582-584.

180. Erlinger, S., Dhumeaux, D. & Benhamou, J.-P. (1969). Effect on bile formation of inhibitors of sodium transport. *Nature, Lond.* 233, 1276-1277.

181. Evrard, E. & Janssen, G. (1968). Gas-liquid chromatographic determination of human fecal bile acids. *J. Lipid. Res.* 9, 226-236.

182. Fahrenbach, M. J., Riccardi, B. A. & Grant, W. C. (1966). Hypocholesterolemic activity of mucilaginous polysaccharides in white leghorn cockerels. *Proc. Soc. exp. Biol. Med.* 123, 321-326.

183. Fallon, J. H. & Woods, J. W. (1968). Response of hyperlipoproteinemia to cholestyramine resin. *J. Am. med. Ass.* 204, 1161-1164.

184. Faloon, W. W., Paes, I. C., Woolfolk, D., Nankin, H., Wallace, K. & Haro, E. N. (1966). Effect of neomycin and kanamycin upon intestinal absorption. *Ann. N.Y. Acad. Sci.* 132, 879-897.

185. Feldman, D. S., Rabinovitch, S. & Feldman, E. B. (1971). Effects of bile salts and detergents on ion transport of absorbing jejunum. *J. clin. Invest.* 50, 29A (abstract).

186. Fiasse, R., Eyssen, R., Dive, C., Harvengt, C., Kestens, P. J. & Nagant de Deuxchaisnes, C. (1970). Metabolism of bile acids, lipids and calcium in Crohn's disease with and without resection. *4th World Congress of Gastroenterology. Copenhagen 1970. Advance abstracts,* p. 354.

187. Fields, M. & Duthie, H. L. (1965). Effect of vagotomy on intraluminal digestion of fat in man. *Gut* 6, 301-310.

188. Fieser, L. F. & Fieser, M. (1959). *Steroids.* New York: Reinhold.

189. Fisher, M. M. & Miyai, K. (1971). Lithocholic acid induced intrahepatic cholestasis. *Gastroenterology* 60, 193 (abstract).

190. Floch, M. H., Gershengoren, W., Elliott, S. & Spiro, H. M. (1971). Bile acid inhibition of the intestinal microflora—a function for simple bile acids? *Gastroenterology* 61, 228-233.

191. Fordtran, J. S. & Locklear, T. W. (1966). Ionic constituents and osmolality of gastric and small intestinal fluids after eating. *Am. J. dig. Dis.* 11, 503-521.

192. Fordtran, J. S., Soergel, K. H. & Ingelfinger, F. J. (1961). Intestinal absorption of D-xylose in man. *New Engl. J. Med.* 267, 274-279.

193. Forell, M. M., Otte, M., Kohl, H. J., Lehnert, P. & Stahlheber, H. P. (1971). The influence of bile and pure bile salts on pancreatic secretion in man. *Scand. J. Gastroent.* 6, 261-266.

194. Forman, D. T., Garvin, J. E., Forestner, J. E. & Taylor, C. B. (1968). Increased excretion of fecal bile acids by an oral hydrophilic colloid. *Proc. Soc. exp. Biol. Med.* 127, 1060-1063.

195. Forsgren, L. (1969). Studies on the intestinal absorption of labelled fat-soluble vitamins (A, D, E and K) via the thoracic duct lymph in the absence of bile in man. *Acta chir. scand. Suppl.* 399.

196. Forth, W. & Glasner, H. (1968). Zur resorption freier und konjugierter Gallensäuren im Dünndarm der Ratte *in vitro* und *in vivo. Arch. exp. Path. Pharmak.* 261, 314-328.

197. Forth, W., Rummel, W. & Glasner, H. (1966). Zur resorptions-hemmenden Wirkung von Gallensäuren. *Arch. exp. Path. Pharmak.* 254, 364-380.

198. Frazer, A. C. (1946). The absorption of triglyceride fat from the intestine. *Physiol. Rev.* 26, 103-119.

199. Frazer, A. C. & Sammons, H. J. (1945). The formation of mono- and di-glycerides during the hydrolysis of triglyceride by pancreatic lipase. *Biochem. J.* 39, 122-128.

200. Frazer, A. C., Schulman, J. H. & Stewart, H. C. (1944). Emulsification of fat in the intestine of the rat and its relationship to absorption. *J. Physiol.* 103, 306-316.

201. Freimuth, U., Zawta, B. & Büchner, M. (1967). Ein neues chromatographisches System zur Trennung strukturisomerer freier Gallensäuren. *J. Chromatog.* 30, 607-610.

202. Frölicher, E. (1936). Die Resorption von Gallensäuren aus verschiedenen Dünndarmabschnitten. *Biochem. Z.* **283**, 273-279.

203. Fromm, H. & Hofmann, A. F. (1971). Breath test for altered bile-acid metabolism. *Lancet* **2**, 621-625.

204. Frosch, B. & Wagener, H. (1967). Quantitative determination of conjugated bile acids in serum in acute hepatitis. *Nature, Lond.* **213**, 404-405.

205. Fry, R. J. M. & Staffeldt, E. (1964). Effect of a diet containing sodium deoxycholate on the intestinal mucosa of the mouse. *Nature, Lond.* **203**, 1396-1398.

206. Fürth, O. & Minnibeck, H. (1931). Über das Mengenverhältnis von Gallensäuren und Fetten im Darminhalte und dessen Beziehung zur Fettresorption. *Biochem. Z.* **237**, 139-158.

207. Galapeaux, E. A., Templeton, R. D. & Borkon, E. L. (1938). The influence of bile on the motility of the dog's colon. *Am. J. Physiol.* **121**, 130-136.

208. Gallo, D. G., Bailey, K. R. & Sheffner, A. L. (1965). The interaction between cholestyramine and drugs. *Proc. Soc. exp. Biol. Med.* **120**, 60-65.

209. Gallo-Torres, H. E., Miller, O. N. & Hamilton, J. G. (1969). A comparison of the effect of bile salts on the absorption of cholesterol from the intestine of the rat. *Biochim. biophys. Acta* **176**, 605-615.

210. Gans, J. H. & Cater, M. R. (1968). Effects of catecholamines on bile acid metabolism in dogs. *Fedn Proc.* **27**, 573 (abstract).

211. Gänshirt, H., Koss, F. W. & Morianz, K. (1960). Untersuchung zur quantitativen Auswertung der Dünnschichtchromatographie. 2. Mitteilung: Trennung und Bestimmung von Gallensäuren. *Arzneimittelforsch* **10**, 943-947.

212. Garbutt, J. Heaton, K. W., Lack, L. & Tyor, M. P. (1969). Increased ratio of glycine- to taurine-conjugated bile salts in patients with ileal disorders. *Gastroenterology* **56**, 711-720.

213. Garbutt, J. T., Lack, L. & Tyor, M. P. (1971). Physiological basis of alterations in the relative conjugation of bile acids with glycine and taurine. *Am. J. clin. Nutr.* **24**, 218-228.

214. Garbutt, J. T., Wilkins, R. M., Lack, L. & Tyor, M. P. (1970). Bacterial modification of taurocholate during enterohepatic recirculation in normal man and patients with small intestinal disease. *Gastroenterology* **59**, 553-566.

215. Gasbarrini, G., Bianchi, F. B., Roda, E., DeVecchis, A. & Peta, G. (1968). L'effetto del carico ematico di acido taurolitocolico

sul fegato di ratto. Aspetti morfologici e riflessi in campo di patologia umana. *Arch. Ital. Mal. Appar. Dig.* **35**, 501-512.

216. Gazet, J.-C. & Kopp, J. (1964). The surgical significance of the ileocecal junction. *Surgery, St. Louis* **56**, 565-573.

217. Geall, M. G., Phillips, S. F. & Summerskill, W. H. J. (1970). Profile of gastric potential difference in man. Effects of aspirin, alcohol, bile and endogenous acid. *Gastroenterology* **58**, 437-443.

218. Gear, M. W. L., Truelove, S. C. & Whitehead, R. (1971). Gastric ulcer and gastritis. *Gut* **12**, 639-645.

219. Gibaldi, M. (1970). Role of surface-active agents in drug absorption. *Fedn Proc.* **29**, 1343-1349.

220. Gibson, T. (1684). *The Anatomy of Humane Bodies.* 2nd edn. London: Flesher.

221. Glasser, J. E., Weiner, I. M. & Lack, L. (1965). Comparative physiology of intestinal taurocholate transport. *Am. J. Physiol.* **208**, 359-362.

222. Glisson, F. (1659). *Anatomia Hepatis.* Amsterdam: Ravesteyn.

223. Gmelin, L. (1826). Cited by Strecker, A. (1848).

224. Gorbach, S. L. (1971). Intestinal microflora. *Gastroenterology* **60**, 1110-1129.

225. Gorbach, S. L., Nahas, L., Weinstein, L., Levitan, R. & Patterson, J. F. (1967). Studies of intestinal microflora. IV. The microflora of ileostomy effluent; a unique microbial ecology. *Gastroenterology* **53**, 874-880.

226. Gorbach, S. L., Plaut, A. G., Nahas, L., Weinstein, L., Spanknebel, G. & Levitan, R. (1967). Studies of intestinal microflora. II. Micro organisms of the small intestine and their relations to oral and fecal flora. *Gastroenterology* **53**, 856-867.

227. Gorbach, S. L. & Tabaqchali, S. (1969). Bacteria, bile and the small bowel. *Gut* **10**, 963-972.

228. Gordon, H., Lewis, B., Eales, L. & Brock, J. F. (1957a). Effect of different dietary fats on the faecal end-products of cholesterol metabolism. *Nature, Lond.* **180**, 923-924.

229. Gordon, H., Lewis, B., Eales, L. & Brock, J. F. (1957b). Dietary fat and cholesterol metabolism. Faecal elimination of bile acids and other lipids. *Lancet* **2**, 1299-1306.

230. Gordon, S. G. & Kern, F. (1968). The absorption of bile salts and fatty acids by hamster small intestine. *Biochim. biophys. Acta* **152**, 372-378.

231. Gordon, S. G. & Kern, F. (1970). The effect of taurocholate on jejunal glyceride synthesis. *Gastroenterology* **58**, 953 (abstract).

232. Gottfries, A. (1969). Lysolecithin: a factor in the pathogenesis of acute cholecystitis? *Acta chir. scand.* **135**, 213-217.

233. Gracey, M. (1971). Intestinal absorption in the 'contaminated small-bowel syndrome'. *Gut* **12**, 403-410.

234. Gracey, M., Burke, V. & Oshin, A. (1971). Influence of bile salts on intestinal sugar transport *in vivo. Scand. J. Gastroent.* **6**, 273-276.

235. Gracey, M., Burke, V., Oshin, A., Barker, J. & Glasgow, E. F. (1971). Bacteria, bile salts and intestinal monosaccharide absorption. *Gut* **12**, 683-692.

236. Grant, R., Grossman, M. I. & Ivy, A. C. (1948). Effect of bile on gastric mucus. *Am. J. Physiol.* **155**, 440 (abstract).

237. Greaves, J. D. & Schmidt, C. L. A. (1933). The rôle played by bile in the absorption of vitamin D in the rat. *J. biol. Chem.* **102**, 101-112.

238. Greene, C. H., Aldrich, M. & Rowntree, L. G. (1928). Studies in the metabolism of the bile. III. The enterohepatic circulation of the bile acids. *J. biol. Chem.* **80**, 753-760.

239. Gregg, J. A. (1966). New solvent systems for thin-layer chromatography of bile acids. *J. Lipid Res.* **7**, 579-581.

240. Gregg, J. A. (1967). Presence of bile acids in jaundiced human urine. *Nature, Lond.* **214**, 29-31.

241. Greim, H. & Popper, H. (1971). Hepatic bile acids after bile duct ligation in rats. *Fedn Proc.* **30**, 634 (abstract).

242. Griffen, W. O., Richardson, J. D. & Medley, E. S. (1970). Prevention of small bowel contamination by ileocecal valve. *Gastroenterology* **58**, 956 (abstract).

243. Gross, L. & Brotman, M. (1970). Hypoprothrombinemia and hemorrhage associated with cholestyramine therapy. *Ann. intern. Med.* **72**, 95-96.

244. Grundy, S. M. & Ahrens, E. H. (1969). Measurements of cholesterol turnover, synthesis and absorption in man, carried out by isotope kinetic and sterol balance methods. *J. Lipid Res.* **10**, 91-107.

245. Grundy, S. M. & Ahrens, E. H. (1970). The effects of unsaturated dietary fats on absorption, excretion, synthesis, and distribution of cholesterol in man. *J. clin. Invest.* **49**, 1135-1152.

245a. Grundy, S. M., Ahrens, E. H. & Davignon, J. (1969). The interaction of cholesterol absorption and cholesterol synthesis in man. *J. Lipid Res.* **10**, 304-315.

246. Grundy, S. M., Ahrens, E. H. & Miettinen, T. A. (1965). Quantitative isolation and gas-liquid chromatographic analysis of total fecal bile acids. *J. Lipid Res.* **6**, 397-410.

247. Grundy, S. M., Ahrens, E. H. & Salen, G. (1968). Dietary β-sitosterol as an internal standard to correct for cholesterol losses in sterol balance studies. *J. Lipid Res.* **9**, 374-387.

248. Grundy, S. M., Ahrens, E. H. & Salen, G. (1971). Interruption of the enterohepatic circulation of bile acids in man: comparative effects of cholestyramine and ileal exclusion on cholesterol metabolism. *J. Lab. clin. Med.* **78**, 94-121.

249. Grundy, S. M., Hofmann, A. F., Davignon, J. & Ahrens, E. H. (1966). Human cholesterol synthesis is regulated by bile acids. *J. clin. Invest.* **45**, 1018-1019 (abstract).

250. Grütte, F. K. & Gärtner, H. (1969). Dünnschicht chromatographische Trennung der Gallensäuren, insbesondere der freien Dihydroxycholansäuren. *J. Chromatog.* **41**, 132-135.

251. Gustafsson, B. E., Bergström, S., Lindstedt, S. & Norman, A. (1957). Turnover and nature of fecal bile acids in germfree and infected rats fed cholic acid-24-[14]C. *Proc. Soc. exp. Biol. Med.* **94**, 467-471.

252. Gustafsson, B. E., Midtvedt, T. & Norman, A. (1966). Isolated fecal micro organisms capable of 7α-dehydroxylating bile acids. *J. exp. Med.* **123**, 413-432.

253. Gustafsson, B. E., Midtvedt, T. & Norman, A. (1968). Metabolism of cholic acid in germfree animals after the establishment in the intestinal tract of deconjugating and 7α-dehydroxylating bacteria. *Acta path. microbiol. scand.* **72**, 433-443.

254. Gustafsson, B. E. & Norman, A. (1962). Comparison of bile acids in intestinal contents of germfree and conventional rats. *Proc. Soc. exp. Biol. Med.* **110**, 387-389.

255. Gustafsson, B. E. & Norman, A. (1968). Physical state of bile acids in intestinal contents of germfree and conventional rats. *Scand. J. Gastroent.* **3**, 625-631.

256. Gustafsson, B. E. & Norman, A. (1969a). Influence of the diet on the turnover of bile acids in germ-free and conventional rats. *Br. J. Nutr.* **23**, 429-442.

257. Gustafsson, B. E. & Norman, A. (1969b). Bile acid absorption from the caecal contents of germ-free rats. *Scand. J. Gastroent.* **4**, 585-590.

258. Gustafsson, B. E., Norman, A. & Sjövall, J. (1960). Influence of *E.coli* infection on turnover and metabolism of cholic acid in germ-free rats. *Archs Biochem. Biophys.* **91**, 93-100.

259. Gutstein, S., Alpert, S. & Arias, I. M. (1968). Studies of hepatic excretory function. IV. Biliary excretion of sulfobromophthalein sodium in a patient with the Dubin-Johnson syndrome and a biliary fistula. *Israel J. med. Sci.* **4**, 36-40.

260. Hadorn, B., Steiner, N., Sumida, C. & Peters, T. J. (1971). Intestinal enterokinase. Mechanisms of its 'secretion' into the lumen of the small intestine. *Lancet* **1**, 165-166.

261. Hagerman, L. M., Cook, D. A. & Schneider, D. L. (1971). *In vitro* binding of taurine- and glycine-conjugated bile salts by cholestyramine. *Fedn Proc.* **30**, 344 (abstract).

262. Hallion, L. & Nepper, H. (1907). Cited by Sobotka (1937).

263. Hamilton, J. D. (1971). The absorption of oleic acid from emulsion and micellar solution. *Biochim. biophys. Acta* **239**, 1-8.

264. Hamilton, J. D., Dyer, N. H., Dawson, A. M., O'Grady, F. W., Vince, A., Fenton, J. C. B. & Mollin, D. L. (1970). Assessment and significance of bacterial overgrowth in the small bowel. *Q. Jl Med.* **39**, 265-285.

265. Hamilton, J. G. (1963). The effect of oral neomycin on the conversion of cholic acid to deoxycholic in man. *Archs Biochem. Biophys.* **101**, 7-13.

266. Hansson, K. (1967). Experimental and clinical studies in aetiologic role of bile reflux in acute pancreatitis. *Acta chir. scand. Supp.* 375.

267. Hansson, K., Lundh, G., Stenram, U. & Wallerström, A. (1963). Pancreatitis and free bile acids. *Acta chir. scand.* **126**, 338-345.

268. Hardison, W. G. (1971). Metabolism of sodium dehydrocholate by the rat liver: its effect on micelle formation in bile. *J. Lab. clin. Med.* **77**, 811-820.

269. Hardison, W. G. M. & Francis, T. I. (1969). The mechanism of cholesterol and phospholipid excretion in bile. *Gastroenterology* **56**, 1164 (abstract).

270. Hardison, W. G. M. & Rosenberg, I. H. (1967). Bile-salt deficiency in the steatorrhea following resection of the ileum and proximal colon. *New Engl. J. Med.* **277**, 337-342.

271. Hartley, G. S. (1936). *Aqueous Solutions of Paraffin-chain Salts. A Study in Micelle Formation.* Paris: Hermann.

272. Hashim, S. A., Bergen, S. S. & van Itallie, T. B. (1961). Experimental steatorrhea induced in man by bile acid sequestrant. *Proc. Soc. exp. Biol. Med.* **106**, 173-175.

273. Hashim, S. A. & van Itallie, T. B. (1965). Cholestyramine resin therapy for hypercholesterolemia. *J. Am. med. Ass.* **192**, 289-293.

274. Haslewood, G. A. D. (1967a). Bile salt evolution. *J. Lipid Res.* **8**, 535-550.
275. Haslewood, G. A. D. (1967b). *Bile Salts.* London: Methuen.
276. Haust, H. L. & Beveridge, J. M. R. (1958). Effect of varying type and quantity of dietary fat on the fecal excretion of bile acids in humans subsisting on formula diets. *Archs Biochem. Biophys.* **78**, 367-375.
277. Heath, T., Caple, I. W. & Redding, P. M. (1970). Effect of the enterohepatic circulation of bile salts on the flow of bile and its content of bile salts and lipids in sheep. *Q. Jl exp. Physiol.* **55**, 93-103.
278. Heaton, K. W. (1968). *The Role of the Distal Small Intestine in the Enterohepatic Circulation of the Conjugated Bile Acids.* M.D. Dissertation, Cambridge.
279. Heaton, K. W. (1969). The importance of keeping bile salts in their place. *Gut* **10**, 857-863.
280. Heaton, K. W., Austad, W. I., Lack, L. & Tyor, M. P. (1968). Enterohepatic circulation of C^{14}-labelled bile salts in disorders of the distal small bowel. *Gastroenterology* **55**, 5-16.
281. Heaton, K. W, & Heaton, S. T. (1970). Unpublished observations.
282. Heaton, K. W., Heaton, S. T. & Barry, R. E. (1971). An *in vivo* comparison of two bile salt-binding agents, cholestyramine and lignin. *Scand. J. Gastroent.* **6**, 281-286.
283. Heaton, K. W. & Lack, L. (1968). Ileal bile salt transport: mutual inhibition in an *in vivo* system. *Am. J. Physiol.* **214**, 585-590.
284. Heaton, K. W., Lever, J. V. & Barnard, D. (1972). Osteomalacia associated with cholestyramine therapy for post-ileectomy diarrhea. *Gastroenterology* **62**, 642-646.
285. Heaton, K. W. & Read, A. E. (1969). Gallstones in patients with disorders of the terminal ileum and disturbed bile salt metabolism. *Br. Med. J.* **3**, 494-496.
286. Hegardt, F. G. & Dam, H. (1971). The solubility of cholesterol in aqueous solutions of bile salts and lecithin. *Z. Ernährungsw.* **10**, 223-233.
287. Hellström, K. (1965). On the bile acid and neutral fecal steroid excretion in man and rabbits following cholesterol feeding. *Acta physiol. scand.* **63**, 21-35.
288. Hellström, K. & Lindstedt, S. (1964). Cholic-acid turnover and biliary bile-acid composition in humans with abnormal thyroid function. *J. Lab. clin. Med.* **63**, 666-679.
289. Hellström, K. & Lindstedt, S. (1966). Studies on the formation of cholic acid in subjects given standardised diet with butter or corn oil as dietary fat. *Am. J. clin. Nutr.* **18**, 46-59.

290. Hellström, K. & Sjövall, J. (1961a). On the origin of lithocholic and ursodeoxycholic acids in man. *Acta physiol. scand.* 51, 218-223.

291. Hellström, K. & Sjövall, J. (1961b). Conjugation of bile acids in patients with hypothyroidism. *J. Atheroscler. Res.* 1, 205-210.

292. Hellström, K. & Sjövall, J. (1962). Turnover of deoxycholic acid in the rabbit. *J. Lipid Res.* 3, 397-404.

293. Hellström, K., Sjövall, J. & Wigand, G. (1962). Influence of semi-synthetic diet and type of fat on the turnover of deoxycholic acid in the rabbit. *J. Lipid Res.* 3, 405-412.

294. Hellström, K. & Strand, O. (1963). Effects of adrenalectomy and corticoid replacement on bile acid conjugation in bile fistula rats. *Acta endocr. Copenh.* 43, 305-310.

294a. Hepner, G. W., Thomas, P. J. & Hofmann, A. F. (1972). Measurement of bile-acid deconjugation in healthy man: metabolism of the steroid and amino acid moieties of cholyl glycine (glycocholic acid). *Gastroenterology* 62, 189 (abstract).

295. Hikasa, Y., Matsuda, S., Nagase, M. *et al.* (1969). Initiating factors of gallstones, especially cholesterol stones (III). *Arch. jap. Chir.* 38, 107-124.

296. Hill, M. J., Crowther, J. S., Drasar, B. S., Hawksworth, G., Aries, V. & Williams, R. E. O. (1971). Bacteria and aetiology of cancer of large bowel. *Lancet* 1, 95-100.

297. Hill, M. J. & Drasar, B. S. (1968). Degradation of bile salts by human intestinal bacteria. *Gut* 9, 22-27.

298. Hislop, I. G., Hofmann, A. F. & Schoenfield, L. J. (1967). Determinants of the rate and site of bile acid absorption in man. *J. clin. Invest.* 46, 1070-1071 (abstract).

299. Hoffmann, H. (1844). Verdauungslehre. *Arch. ges Med.* 6, 157-188.

300. Hoffman, N. E., Simmonds, W. J. & Morgan, R. G. H. (1971). A comparison of absorption of free fatty acid and α-glyceryl ether in the presence and absence of a micellar phase. *Biochim. biophys. Acta* 231, 487-495.

301. Hofmann, A. F. (1962). Thin-layer adsorption chromatography of free and conjugated bile acids on silicic acid. *J. Lipid Res.* 3, 127-128.

302. Hofmann, A. F. (1963). The function of bile salts in fat absorption. *Biochem. J.* 89, 57-68.

303. Hofmann, A. F. (1964). Thin-layer chromatography of the bile acids and their derivatives. in *New Biochemical Separations,*

ed. James, A. T. & Morris, L. J., pp. 262-282. Princeton: van Nostrand.

304. Hofmann, A. F. (1965). Clinical implications of physicochemical studies on bile salts. *Gastroenterology* **48**, 484-494.

305. Hofmann, A. F. (1966). A physicochemical approach to the intraluminal phase of fat absorption. *Gastroenterology* **50**, 56-64.

306. Hofmann, A. F. (1967). The syndrome of ileal disease and the broken enterohepatic circulation: cholerheic enteropathy. *Gastroenterology* **52**, 752-757.

307. Hofmann, A. F. (1968). Functions of bile in the alimentary canal. In *Handbook of Physiology,* Section 6: Alimentary Canal, Vol. V: Bile; digestion; ruminal physiology, ed. Code, C. F., pp. 2507-2533. Washington: American Physiological Society.

308. Hofmann, A. F. (1970). Gastroenterology: physical events in lipid digestion and absorption. Introductory remarks. *Fedn Proc.* **29**, 1317-1319.

309. Hofmann, A. F. & Borgström, B. (1962). Physico-chemical state of lipids in intestinal content during their digestion and absorption. *Fedn Proc.* **21**, 43-50.

310. Hofmann, A. F. & Borgström, B. (1964). The intraluminal phase of fat digestion in man: the lipid content of the micellar and oil phases of intestinal content obtained during fat digestion and absorption. *J. clin. Invest.* **43**, 247-257.

311. Hofmann, A. F. & Mosbach, E. H. (1964). Identification of allodeoxycholic acid as the major component of gallstones induced in the rabbit by 5α-cholestan-3β-ol. *J. biol. Chem.* **239**, 2813-2821.

312. Hofmann, A. F. & Poley, J. R. (1969). Cholestyramine treatment of diarrhea associated with ileal resection. *New Engl. J. Med.* **281**, 397-402.

313. Hofmann, A. F., Schoenfield, L. J., Kottke, B. A. & Poley, J. R. (1970). Methods for the description of bile acid kinetics in man. In *Methods in Medical Research,* Vol. 12, ed. Olson, R. E., pp. 149-180. Chicago: Year Book Medical Publishers.

314. Hofmann, A. F. & Small, D. M. (1967). Detergent properties of bile salts: correlation with physiological function. *A. Rev. Med.* **18**, 333-376.

315. Hofmann, A. F., Thomas, P. J., Smith, L. H. & McCall, J. T. (1970). Pathogenesis of secondary hyperoxaluria in patients with ileal resection and diarrhea. *Gastroenterology* **58**, 960 (abstract).

316. Holsti, P. (1956). Experimental cirrhosis of the liver in rabbits induced by gastric instillation of desiccated whole bile. *Acta path. microbiol. scand. Supp.* 113, 1-67.

317. Holsti, P. (1960). Cirrhosis of the liver induced in rabbits by gastric instillation of 3-monohydroxycholanic acid. *Nature, Lond.* 186, 250.

318. Holsti, P. (1962).Bile acids as a cause of liver injury. Cirrhogenic effect of chenodesoxycholic acid in rabbits. *Acta path. microbiol. scand.* 54, 479.

319. Holt, P. R. (1964). Intestinal absorption of bile salts in the rat. *Am. J. Physiol.* 207, 1-7.

320. Holt, P. R. (1966). Competitive inhibition of intestinal bile salt absorption in the rat. *Am. J. Physiol.* 210, 635-639.

321. Holzbach, R. T. & Marsh, M. (1971). Definition of cholesterol solubility in human bile. *Gastroenterology* 60, 677 (abstract).

322. Holzbach, R. T., Marsh, M. & Holan, K. (1971). Cholesterol solubilising capacity: a direct assessment of lithogenic potential in bile. *Gastroenterology* 60, 777 (abstract).

323. Hoppe-Seyler, F. (1863). Ueber die Schicksale der Galle in Darmkanale. *Virchows Arch. path. Anat. Physiol.* 26, 519-537.

324. Horrall, O. H. (1938). *Bile: its Toxicity and Relation to Disease.* University of Chicago Press.

325. Howard, A. N. & Hyams, D. E. (1971). Combined use of clofibrate and cholestyramine or DEAE Sephadex in hypercholesterolaemia. *Br. med. J.* 3, 25-27.

326. Howell, J. I., Lucy, J. A., Pirola, R. C. & Bouchier, I. A. D. (1970). Macromolecular assemblies of lipid in bile. *Biochim. biophys. acta* 210, 1-6.

327. Hunt, R. D. (1965). Proliferation of bile ductules (the ductular cell reaction) induced by lithocholic acid. *Fedn Proc.* 24, 431 (abstract).

328. Hunt, R. D., Leveille, G. A. & Sauberlich, H. E. (1964). Dietary bile acids and lipid metabolism. III. Effects of lithocholic acid in mammalian species. *Proc. Soc. exp. Biol. Med.* 115, 277-280.

329. Irvin, J. L., Johnston, C. G. & Kopala, J. (1944). A photometric method for the determination of cholates in bile and blood. *J. biol. Chem.* 153, 439-457.

330. Irvin, J. L., Johnston, C. G. & Sharp, E. A. (1946). The enterohepatic circulation of foreign bile acids: the circulation of cholates in hogs with biliary fistulae. *Am. J. Physiol.* 146, 293-306.

331. Isaksson, B. (1954). A method for spectrophotometric determination of chenodesoxycholic acid in bile. *Acta chem. scand.* **8**, 889-897.

332. Ivey, K. J. (1971). Gastric mucosal barrier. *Gastroenterology* **61**, 246-257.

333. Ivey, K. J., DenBesten, L. & Bell, S. (1970). Absorption of bile salts from the human stomach. *J. appl. Physiol.* **29**, 806-808.

334. Ivey, K. J., DenBesten, L. & Clifton, J. A. (1970). Effect of bile salts on ionic movement across the human gastric mucosa. *Gastroenterology* **59**, 683-690.

335. Iwata, T. & Yamasaki, K. (1964). Enzymatic determination and thin-layer chromatography of bile acids in blood. *J. Biochem.* **56**, 424-431.

336. Izumi, K. (1965). Studies on the chemical composition of gallbladder bile and gallstone; especially on the difference between cholesterol stone and pigment stone. *Fukuoka Acta med.* **56**, 488-523.

337. Jacobsen, J. G. & Smith, L. H. (1968). Biochemistry and physiology of taurine and taurine derivatives. *Physiol. Rev.* **48**, 424-511.

338. Javitt, N. B. (1969). Bile salt regulation of hepatic excretory function. *Gastroenterology* **56**, 622-625.

339. Javitt, N. B. & Emerman, S. (1968). Effect of sodium taurolithocholate on bile flow and bile acid excretion. *J. clin. Invest.* **47**, 1002-1014.

340. Johansson, G. (1970). Effect of cholestyramine and diet on hydroxylations in the biosynthesis and metabolism of bile acids. *Eur. J. Biochem.* **17**, 292-295.

341. Johnston, J. M. & Borgstrom, B. (1964). The intestinal absorption and metabolism of micellar solutions of lipids. *Biochim. biophys. Acta* **84**, 412-423.

342. Jordan, P. H., Olson, R. & Paige, R. (1968). Is the gallbladder's reservoir function important after small bowel resection? *Surgery, St. Louis* **64**, 446-450.

343. Josephson, B. (1941). The circulation of the bile acids in connection with their production, conjugation and excretion. *Physiol. Rev.* **21**, 463-486.

344. Josephson, B. & Rydin, A. (1936). The resorption of the bile acids from the intestines. *Biochem. J.* **30**, 2224-2228.

345. Juniper, K. (1965). Physicochemical characteristics of bile and their relation to gallstone formation. *Am. J. Med.* **39**, 98-107.

346. Kalser, M. H., Roth, J. L. A., Tumen, H. & Johnson, T. A. (1960). Relation of small bowel resection to nutrition in man. *Gastroenterology* **38**, 605-615.

347. Kapadia, C. R., Radhakrishnan, A. N., Mathan, V. I. & Baker, S. J. (1971a). A study of the ratios of bile salt conjugates of glycine to taurine in the jejunum and ileum in patients with tropical sprue. *Scand. J. Gastroent.* **6**, 357-361.

348. Kapadia, C. R., Radhakrishnan, A. N., Mathan, V. I. & Baker, S. J. (1971b). Studies on bile salt deconjugation in patients with tropical sprue. *Scand. J. Gastroent.* **6**, 29-32.

349. Kappas, A. & Palmer, R. H. (1963). Selected aspects of steroid pharmacology. *Pharmac. Rev.* **15**, 123-167.

350. Kayden, H. J., Senior, J. R. & Mattson, F. H. (1967). The monoglyceride pathway of fat absorption in man. *J. clin. Invest.* **46**, 1695-1703.

351. Kaye, M. D., Struthers, J. E., Tidball, J. S., Kern, F. & DeNiro, E. (1971). Metabolism of isotopically labelled cholic acid in cirrhosis. *Gastroenterology* **60**, 186 (abstract).

352. Kellock, T. D., Pearson, J. R., Russell, R. I., Walker, J. G. & Wiggins, H. S. (1969). The incidence and clinical significance of faecal hydroxy fatty acids. *Gut* **10**, 1055 (abstract).

353. Kellogg, T. F., Knight, P. L, & Wostmann, B. S. (1970). Effect of bile acid deconjugation on the fecal excretion of steroids. *J. Lipid Res.* **11**, 362-366.

354. Kenney, T. J. & Garbutt, J. T. (1970). Effect of cholestyramine on bile acid metabolism in normal man. *Gastroenterology* **58**, 966 (abstract).

355. Kern, F. & Borgström, B. (1965). The effect of a conjugated bile salt on oleic acid absorption in the rat. *Gastroenterology* **49**, 623-631.

356. Keys, A., Grande, F. & Anderson, J. T. (1961). Fiber and pectin in the diet and serum cholesterol concentration in man. *Proc. Soc. exp. Biol. Med.* **106**, 555-558.

357. Kim, Y. S. & Spritz, N. (1968). Hydroxy acid excretion in steatorrhea of pancreatic and nonpancreatic origin. *New Engl. J. Med.* **279**, 1424-1426.

358. Kim, Y. S., Spritz, N., Blum, M., Terz, J. & Sherlock, P. (1966). The role of altered bile acid metabolism in the steatorrhea of experimental blind loop. *J. clin. Invest.* **45**, 956-962.

359. King, J. E., Oshiba, S. & Schoenfield, L. J. (1969). Simulation of taurocholate enterohepatic circulation in isolated hamster liver. *Gastroenterology* **56**, 1216 (abstract).

360. King, J. E. & Schoenfield, L. J. (1971). Lithocholate cholestasis in isolated hamster liver. *Gastroenterology* **60**, 189 (abstract).

361. Kirk, R. M. (1970). Experimental gastric ulcers in the rat: the separate and combined effects of vagotomy and bile-duct implantation into the stomach. *Br. J. Surg.* **57**, 521-524.

362. Klaassen, C. D. (1971a). Species differences in the choleretic response to bile salts. *Fedn Proc.* **30**, 447 (abstract).

363. Klaassen, C. D. (1971b). Does bile acid secretion determine canalicular bile production in rats? *Am. J. Physiol.* **220**, 667-673.

364. Knoebel, L. K. & Ryan, J. M. (1963). Digestion and mucosal absorption of fat in normal and bile-deficient dogs. *Am. J. Physiol.* **204**, 509-514.

365. Kodsi, B. E. (1971). Dialysis of gallbladder bile. *Gastroenterology* **60**, 685 (abstract).

366. Kolman, R., Feigenbaum, A. S. & Bauman, J. W. (1970). Bile acids in hypophysectomised rats. *Fedn Proc.* **29**, 629 (abstract).

367. Kottke, B. A. (1969). Differences in bile acid excretion. Primary hypercholesteremia compared to combined hypercholesteremia and hypertriglyceridemia. *Circulation* **40**, 13-20.

368. Kottke, B. A., Wollenweber, J. & Owen, C. A. (1966). Quantitative thin-layer chromatography of free and conjugated cholic acid in human bile and intestinal contents. *J. Chromatog.* **21**, 439-447.

369. Kravetz, R. E. (1964). Etiology of biliary tract disease in southwestern American Indians. Analysis of 105 consecutive cholecystectomies. *Gastroenterology* **46**, 392-398.

370. Kreek, M. J. (1970). Binding of estradiol and other steroids to cholestyramine *in vitro. Fedn Proc.* **29**, 781 (abstract).

371. Kremen, A. J., Linner, J. H. & Nelson, C. H. (1954). An experimental evaluation of the nutritional importance of proximal and distal small intestine. *Ann. Surg.* **140**, 439-448.

372. Krondl, A., Vavrinkova, H. & Michalec, C. (1964). Effect of cholecystectomy on the role of the gallbladder in fat absorption. *Gut* **5**, 607-610.

373. Krone, C. L., Theodor, E., Sleisenger, M. H. & Jeffries, G. H. (1968). Studies on the pathogenesis of malabsorption. Lipid hydrolysis and micelle formation in the intestinal lumen. *Medicine (Baltimore)* **47**, 89-106.

374. Kuksis, A. (1969). Gas chromatography of bile acids. In *Lipid Chromatographic Analysis* ed. Marinetti, G. V., Vol. 2, pp. 215-312. New York: Dekker.

375. Lack, L. & Weiner, I. M. (1961). *In vitro* absorption of bile salts by small intestine of rats and guinea pigs. *Am. J. Physiol.* **200**, 313-317.

376. Lack, L. & Weiner, I. M. (1963a). Intestinal absorption of bile salts and some biological implications. *Fedn Proc.* **22**, 1334-1338.

377. Lack, L. & Weiner, I. M. (1963b). The intestinal action of benzmalecene: the relationship of its hypocholesterolemic effect to active transport of bile salts and other substances. *J. Pharmac. exp. Ther.* **139**, 248-258.

378. Lack, L. & Weiner, I. M. (1966). Intestinal bile salt transport: structure-activity relationships and other properties. *Am. J. Physiol.* **210**, 1142-1152.

379. Lawrence, A. S. C. (1961). Polar interaction in detergency. In *Surface Activity and Detergency,* ed. Durham, K., pp. 158-191. London: MacMillan.

380. Lee, C.-C. & Herrmann, R. G. (1963). Sucrose diet and biliary cholate excretion in rats: with note on procedure for cholate determination. *Arch. int. Pharmacodyn.* **141**, 591-594.

381. Lee, M. J. & Whitehouse, M. W. (1965). Inhibition of electron transport and coupled phosphorylation in liver mitochondria by cholanic (bile) acids and their conjugates. *Biochim. biophys. Acta* **100**, 317-328.

382. Lee, M. J., Parke, D. V. & Whitehouse, M. W. (1965). Regulation of cholesterol catabolism by bile salts and glycyrrhetic acid *in vivo. Proc. Soc. exp. Biol. Med.* **120**, 6-8.

383. Lees, R. S. & Wilson, D. E. (1971). The treatment of hyperlipidemia. *New Engl. J. Med.* **284**, 186-195.

384. Lehmann, C. G. (1851). Cited by Sobotka (1937).

385. Lehmann, C. G. (1855). *Physiological Chemistry.* 2nd edn. Philadelphia: Blanchard & Lea.

386. Lengemann, F. W. & Dobbins, J. W. (1958). The role of bile in calcium absorption. *J. Nutr.* **66**, 45-54.

387. Lenthall, J., Reynolds, T. B. & Donovan, J. (1970). Excessive output of bile in chronic hepatic disease. *Surgery, St. Louis* **130**, 243-253.

388. LeVeen, H. H., Borek, B., Axelrod, D. R. & Johnson, A. (1967). Cause and treatment of diarrhea following resection of the small intestine. *Surgery Gynec. Obstet.* **124**, 766-770.

389. Leveille, G. A., Hunt, R. D. & Sauberlich, H. E. (1964). Dietary bile acids and lipid metabolism. IV. Dietary level of lithocholic acid for chicks. *Proc. Soc. exp. Biol. Med.* **115**, 569-572.

390. Leveille, G. A. & Sauberlich, H. E. (1966). Mechanism of the cholesterol-depressing effect of pectin in the cholesterol-fed rat. *J. Nutr.* **88**, 209-214.

391. Levin, S. J., Irvin, J. L. & Johnston, C. G. (1961). Spectrofluorometric determination of total bile acids in bile. *Anal. Chem.* **33**, 856-860.

392. Levin, S. J. & Johnston, C. G. (1962). Fluorometric determination of serum total bile acids. *J. Lab. clin. Med.* **59**, 681-686.

393. Levin, S. J., Johnston, C. G. & Boyle, A. J. (1961). Spectrophotometric determination of several bile acids as conjugates. Extraction with ethyl acetate. *Anal. Chem.* **33**, 1407-1411.

394. Lewis, B., Panveliwalla, D., Tabaqchali, S. & Wootton, I. D. P. (1969). Serum-bile-acids in the stagnant-loop syndrome. *Lancet* **1**, 219-220.

395. Liebig, J. (1843). *Animal Chemistry, or Chemistry in its Applications to Physiology and Pathology.* 2nd edn. London: Taylor & Watton.

396. Lin, T. H., Rubinstein, R. & Holmes, W. L. (1963). A study of the effect of D- and L-triiodothyronine on bile acid excretion of rats. *J. Lipid Res.* **4**, 63-67.

397. Lind, L. R. (1969). Translator of *The Epitome of Andreas Vesalius*, p. 44. Cambridge, Massachusetts: M.I.T. Press.

398. Lindsey, C. A. & Wilson, J. D. (1965). Evidence for a contribution by the intestinal wall to the serum cholesterol of the rat. *J. Lipid Res.* **6**, 173-181.

399. Lindstedt, S. (1957a). The turnover of cholic acid in man. *Acta physiol. scand.* **40**, 1-9.

400. Lindstedt, S. (1957b). The formation of deoxycholic acid from cholic acid in man. *Ark. Kemi* **11**, 145-150.

401. Lindstedt, S. & Ahrens, E. H. (1961). Conversion of cholesterol to bile acids in man. *Proc. Soc. exp. Biol. Med.* **108**, 286-288.

402. Lindstedt, S., Avigan, J., Goodman, D. S., Sjövall, J. & Steinberg, D. (1965). The effect of dietary fat on the turnover of cholic acid and on the composition of the biliary bile acids in man. *J. clin. Invest.* **44**, 1754-1765.

403. Lindstedt, S. & Norman, A. (1956a). The turnover of bile acids in the rat. *Acta physiol. scand.* **38**, 121-128.

404. Lindstedt, S. & Norman, A. (1956b). The excretion of bile acids in rats treated with chemotherapeutics. *Acta physiol. scand.* **38**, 129-134.

405. Lindstedt, S. & Samuelsson, B. (1959). On the interconversion of cholic and deoxycholic acid in the rat. *J. biol. Chem.* **234**, 2026-2030.

406. Lipkin, M. (1971). Progress Report. In 'defence' of the gastric mucosa. *Gut* **12**, 599-603.

407. Longenecker, J. B. & Basu, S. G. (1965). Effect of cholestyramine on absorption of amino acids and vitamin A in man. *Fedn Proc.* **24**, 375 (abstract).

408. Lorentz, T. G. (1966). Observations on the pathogenesis of gall-stones. *Br. J. Surg.* **53**, 503-509.

409. Losowsky, M. S. & Walker, B. E. (1969). Liver disease and malabsorption. *Gastroenterology* **56**, 589-600.

410. Low-Beer, T. S., Heaton, K. W., Heaton, S. T. & Read, A. E. (1971). Gallbladder inertia and sluggish enterohepatic circulation of bile-salts in coeliac disease. *Lancet* **1**, 991-994.

411. Low-Beer, T. S., Lack, L. & Tyor, M. P. (1969a). Effect of one meal on enterohepatic circulation of bile salts. *Gastroenterology* **56**, 1179 (abstract).

411a. Low-Beer, T. S., Pomare, E. & Morris, J. S. (1972). The control of bile salt synthesis in man. *Nature, Lond.* (in press).

412. Low-Beer, T. S., Schneider, R. E. & Dobbins, W. O. (1970). Morphological changes of the small-intestinal mucosa of guinea pig and hamster following incubation *in vitro* and perfusion *in vivo* with unconjugated bile salts. *Gut* **11**, 486-492.

413. Low-Beer, T. S., Tyor, M. P. & Lack, L. (1969b). Effect of sulfation of taurolithocholic and glycolithocholic acids on their intestinal transport. *Gastroenterology* **56**, 721-726.

414. McBain, J. W. (1913). Mobility of highly-charged micelles. *Trans. Faraday Soc.* **9**, 99-101.

415. McBain, J. W., Merrill, R. C. & Vinograd, J. R. (1941). The solubilisation of water-insoluble dye in dilute solutions of aqueous detergents. *J. Am. chem. Soc.* **63**, 670-676.

416. McCloy, R. M. & Hofmann, A. F. (1971). Tropical diarrhea in Vietnam—a controlled study of cholestyramine therapy. *New Engl. J. Med.* **284**, 139-140.

417. McCutcheon, A. D. (1968). A fresh approach to the pathogenesis of pancreatitis. *Gut* **9**, 296-310.

418. McIntyre, N. (1971). Sterol absorption—from lumen to liver. *Gut* **12**, 411-416.

419. McLeod, G. M. & Wiggins, H. S. (1968). Bile-salts in small intestinal contents after ileal resection and in other malabsorption syndromes. *Lancet* **1**, 873-876.

420. Macarol, V., Morris, T. Q., Baker, K. J. & Bradley, S. E. (1970). Hydrocortisone choleresis in the dog. *J. clin. Invest.* **49**, 1714-1723.

421. Makino, I., Nakagawa, S. & Mashimo, K. (1969). Conjugated and unconjugated serum bile acid levels in patients with hepatobiliary diseases. *Gastroenterology* **56**, 1033-1039.

421a. Makino, I., Sjövall, J., Norman, A. & Strandvik, B. (1971). Excretion of 3β-hydroxy-5-cholenoic and 3α-hydroxy-5α-cholanoic acids in urine of infants with biliary atresia. *FEBS Letters* **15**, 161.

422. Makita, M. & Wells, W. W. (1963). Quantitative analysis of fecal bile acids by gas-liquid chromatography. *Anal. Biochem.* **5**, 523-530.

423. Mallory, A., Smith, J., Kern, F. & Savage, D. (1971). Patterns of bile acids and microflora in the human small intestine. *Gastroenterology* **60**, 694 (abstract).

424. Marcet, W. (1858). On the action of bile upon fats; with additional observations on excretine. *Proc. roy. Soc. (London)* **9**, 306-308.

425. Marin, G. A., Clark, M. L. & Senior, J. R. (1969). Studies of malabsorption occurring in patients with Laennec's cirrhosis. *Gastroenterology* **56**, 727-736.

426. Meihoff, W. E. & Kern, F. (1968). Bile salt malabsorption in regional ileitis, ileal resection and mannitol-induced diarrhea. *J. clin. Invest.* **47**, 261-267.

427. Mekhjian, H. S. & Phillips, S. F. (1970). Perfusion of the canine colon with unconjugated bile acids. Effect on water and electrolyte transport, morphology and bile acid absorption. *Gastroenterology* **59**, 120-129.

428. Mekhjian, H. S., Phillips, S. F. & Hofmann, A. F. (1971). Colonic secretion of water and electrolytes induced by bile acids: perfusion studies in man. *J. clin. Invest.* **50**, 1569-1577.

429. Mekhjian, H. S., Phillips, S. F. & Hofmann, A. F. (1968). Conjugated bile salts block water and electrolyte transport by the human colon. *Gastroenterology* **54**, 1256 (abstract).

430. Melmon, K. L., Sjoerdsma, A., Oates, J. A. & Laster, L. (1965). Treatment of malabsorption and diarrhea of the carcinoid syndrome with methysergide. *Gastroenterology* **48**, 18-24.

431. Meyer, A. E. & McEwen, J. P. (1948). Bile acids and their choline salts applied to the inner surface of the isolated colon and ileum of the guinea pig. *Am. J. Physiol.* **153**, 386-392.

432. Midtvedt, T. & Norman, A. (1967). Bile acid transformations by microbial strains belonging to genera found in intestinal contents. *Acta path. microbiol. scand.* **71**, 629-638.

433. Midtvedt, T. & Norman, A. (1968a). Parameters in 7α-dehydroxylation of bile acids by anaerobic lactobacilli. *Acta path. microbiol. scand.* **72**, 313-329.

434. Midtvedt, T. & Norman, A. (1968b). Anaerobic, bile acid transforming microorganisms in rat intestinal content. *Acta path. microbiol. scand.* **72**, 337-344.

435. Midtvedt, T., Norman, A. & Nygaard, K. (1970). Metabolism of glycocholic acid in gastrectomised patients. *Scand. J. Gastroent.* **5**, 237-240.

436. Miettinen, T. A. (1971). The role of bile salts in diarrhoea of patients with ulcerative colitis. *Gut* **12**, 632-635.

437. Miettinen, T. A., Pelkonen, R., Nikkilä, E. A. & Heinonen, O. (1967). Low excretion of fecal bile acids in a family with hypercholesterolemia. *Acta med. scand.* **182**, 645-650.

438. Miettinen, T. A. & Peltokallio, P. (1971). Bile salt, fat, water and vitamin B_{12} excretion after ileostomy. *Scand. J. Gastroent.* **6**, 543-552.

439. Miettinen, T. A. & Siurala, M. (1971). Micellar solubilisation of intestinal lipids and sterols in gluten enteropathy and liver cirrhosis. *Scand. J. Gastroent.* **6**, 527-535.

440. Mishkin, S. & Kessler, J. I. (1970). The uptake and release of bile salt and fatty acid by hamster jejunum. *Biochim. biophys. Acta* **202**, 222-224.

441. Mitropoulos, K. A. & Myant, N. B. (1967). The formation of lithocholic acid, chenodeoxycholic acid and α- and β-muricholic acids from cholesterol incubated with rat-liver mitochondria. *Biochem. J.* **103**, 472-479.

443. Modai, M. & Theodor, E. (1970). Intestinal contents in patients with viral hepatitis after a lipid meal. *Gastroenterology* **58**, 379-387.

444. Moore, B. & Parker, W. H. (1901). On the functions of bile as a solvent. *Proc. roy. Soc. B,* **68**, 64-76.

445. Moore, B, & Rockwood, D. P. (1897). On the mode of absorption of fats. *J. Physiol.* **21**, 58-84.

446. Moore, E. W. & Dietschy, J. M. (1964). Na and K activity coefficients in bile and bile salts determined by glass electrodes. *Am. J. Physiol.* **206**, 1111-1117.

447. Moore, R. B., Anderson, J. T., Taylor, H. L., Keys, A. & Frantz, I. D. (1968). Effect of dietary fat on the fecal excretion of cholesterol and its degradation products in man. *J. clin. Invest.* **47**, 1517-1534.

448. Moore, R. B., Crane, C. A. & Frantz, I. D. (1968). Effect of cholestyramine on the fecal excretion of intravenously administered cholesterol-4-^{14}C and its degradation products in a hypercholesterolemic patient. *J. clin. Invest.* **47**, 1664-1671.

449. Moore, R. B., Frantz, I. D. & Buchwald, H. (1969). Changes in cholesterol pool size, turnover rate and fecal bile acid and sterol excretion after partial ileal bypass in hypercholesteremic patients. *Surgery, St. Louis* **65**, 98-107.

450. Morgan, R. G. H. (1964). The effect of bile salts on the lymphatic absorption by the unanaesthetised rat of intraduodenally infused lipids. *Q. Jl exp. Physiol.* **49**, 457-465.

451. Morgan, R. G. H. & Borgström, B. (1969). The mechanism of fat absorption in the bile fistula rat. *Q. Jl exp. Physiol.* **54**, 228-243.

453. Morris, J. S., Heaton, K. W. & Read, A. E. (1970). Absorption of bile acids by the colon. *Gut* **11**, 1063 (abstract).

454. Morris, J. S., Low-Beer, T. S. & Heaton, K. W. (1971). Unpublished observations.

455. Mosbach, E. H., Abell, L. L. & Halpern, E. (1958). Effect of bile acids and of diet on cholesterol metabolism. *Circulation* **18**, 486 (abstract).

456. Mosbach, E. H., Rothschild, M. A., Abell, L. L. & Oratz, M. (1971). Stimulation of bile acid production by cortisone. *Gastroenterology* **60**, 748 (abstract).

457. Mosbach, E. H., Rothschild, M. A., Bekersky, I., Oratz. M. & Mongelli, J. (1971). Bile acid synthesis in the isolated, perfused rabbit liver. *J. clin. Invest.* **50**, 1720-1730.

458. Moutafis, C. D. & Myant, N. B. (1968). Increased hepatic synthesis of cholesterol after ileal by-pass in monkeys. *Clin. Sci.* **34**, 541-548.

459. Moutafis, C. D. & Myant, N. B. (1969). The metabolism of cholesterol in two hypercholesterolaemic patients treated with cholestyramine. *Clin. Sci.* **37**, 443-454.

460. Mueller, J. H. (1916). The mechanism of cholesterol absorption. *J. biol. Chem.* **27**, 463-480.

461. Murphy, G. M., Billing, B. H. & Baron, D. N. (1970). A fluorimetric and enzymatic method for the estimation of serum total bile acids. *J. clin. Path.* **23**, 594-598.

462. Myant, N. B. & Eder, H. A. (1961). The effect of biliary drainage upon the synthesis of cholesterol in the liver. *J. Lipid Res.* **2**, 363-368.

463. Nahrwold, D. L. & Grossman, M. (1970). Effect of cholecystectomy on bile flow and composition in response to food. *Am. J. Surg.* **119**, 30-34.

464. Nair, P. P., Banwell, J. G., Gorbach, S. L., Lilis, C. & Alcaraz, A. (1970). Tropical sprue and malnutrition in West Bengal. III. Biochemical characteristics of bile salts in the small intestine. *Am. J. clin. Nutr.* **23**, 1569-1578.

465. Nair, P. P. & Garcia, C. (1969). A modified gas-liquid chromatographic procedure for the rapid determination of bile acids in biological fluids. *Anal. Biochem.* **29**, 164-171.

466. Nair, P. P., Garcia-Lilis, C. & Mendeloff, A. I. (1970). Effect of lithocholic acid and antibiotics on tissue bile acids in the rat. *J. Nutr.* **100**, 698-704.

467. Nair, P. P., Gordon, M. & Reback, J. (1967). The enzymatic cleavage of the carbon-nitrogen bond in 3α, 7α, 12α-trihydroxy-5β-cholan-24-oylglycine. *J. biol. Chem.* **242**, 7-11.

467a. Nair, P. P. & Kritchevsky, D. (eds) (1971). *The Bile Acids: Chemistry, Physiology, and Metabolism. Vol. I. Chemistry.* New York: Plenum Press.

468. Nakayama, F. (1971). Studies on calculus versus milieu: gallstone and bile. *J. Lab. clin. Med.* **77**, 366-377.

469. Nakayama, F. & van der Linden, W. (1970). Bile from gallbladder harbouring gallstone: can it indicate stone formation? *Acta chir. scand.* **136**, 605-610.

470. Naqvi, S. H. M., Herndon, B. L., Kelley, M. T., Bleisch, V., Aexel, R. T. & Nicholas, H. J. (1969). Detection of mono-hydroxy 'bile' acids in the brains of guinea pigs afflicted with experimental allergic encephalomyelitis. *J. Lipid Res.* **10**, 115-120.

471. Naqvi, S. H. M., Ramsey, R. B. & Nicholas, H. J. (1970). Detection of lithocholic acid in multiple sclerosis brain tissue. *Lipids* **5**, 578-580.

472. Neale, G., Lewis, B., Weaver, V. & Panveliwalla, D. (1971). Serum bile acids in liver disease. *Gut* **12**, 145-152.

473. Neiderhiser, D. H., Pineda, F. M., Hejduk, L. J. & Roth, H. P. (1971). Absorption of oleic acid by the guinea pig gallbladder. *J. Lab. clin. Med.* **77**, 985-992.

474. Neiderhiser, D. H. & Roth, H. P. (1970). Effect of phospholipase A on cholesterol solubilisation by lecithin in a bile salt solution. *Gastroenterology* **58**, 26-31.

475. Nilsson, S. (1970). Synthesis and secretion of biliary phospholipids in man. *Acta chir. scand. Supp.* **405.**

476. Nilsson, S. & Schers. T. (1969). Importance of bile acids for phospholipid secretion into human hepatic bile. *Gastroenterology* **57,** 525-532.

477. Nilsson, S. & Schersten, T. (1970). Influence of bile acids on the synthesis of biliary phospholipids in man. *Eur. J. clin. Invest.* **1,** 1-13.

478. Nordström, C. & Dahlqvist, A. (1971). Intestinal enterokinase. *Lancet* **1,** 1185-1186 (letter).

479. Norman, A. (1964). Faecal excretion products of cholic acid in man. *Br. J. Nutr.* **18,** 173-186.

480. Norman, A. (1970). Metabolism of glycocholic acid in man. *Scand. J. Gastroent.* **5,** 231-236.

481. Norman, A. & Palmer, R. H. (1964). Metabolites of lithocholic acid-24-C^{14} in human bile and feces. *J. Lab. clin. Med.* **63,** 986-1001.

482. Norman, A. & Shorb, M. S. (1962). *In vitro* formation of deoxycholic and lithocholic acid by human intestinal microorganisms. *Proc. Soc. exp. Biol. Med.* **110,** 552-555.

483. Norman, A. & Sjövall, J. (1958). On the transformation and enterohepatic circulation of cholic acid in the rat. *J. biol. chem.* **233,** 872-885.

484. Norman, A. & Sjövall, J. (1960). Formation of lithocholic acid from chenodeoxycholic acid in the rat. *Acta chem. scand.* **14,** 1815-1818.

485. Norman, A. & Widström, O. A. (1964). Hydrolysis of conjugated bile acids by extracellular enzymes present in rat intestinal contents. *Proc. Soc. exp. biol. Med.* **117,** 442-444.

486. Northfield, T. C., Condillac, E. & McColl, I. (1970). Bile salt metabolism in the normal human small intestine. *Gut* **11,** 1063 (abstract).

487. Oi, M., Oshida, K. & Sugimura, S. (1959). The location of gastric ulcers. *Gastroenterology* **36,** 45-56.

488. Okishio, T. & Nair, P. P. (1966). Studies on bile acids. Some observations on the intracellular localisation of major bile acids in rat liver. *Biochemistry* **5,** 3662-3668.

489. Olivecrona, T. & Sjövall, J. (1959). Bile acids in rat portal blood. *Acta physiol. scand.* **46,** 284-290.

490. Olson, J. A. (1964). The effect of bile and bile salts on the uptake and cleavage of β-carotene into retinol ester (vitamin A ester) by intestinal slices. *J. Lipid Res.* **5,** 402-408.

491. O'Máille, E. R. L., Richards, T. G. & Short, A. H. (1965). Acute taurine depletion and maximal rates of hepatic conjugation and secretion of cholic acid in the dog. *J. Physiol.* **180**, 67-80.

492. O'Máille, E. R. L., Richards, T. G. & Short, A. H. (1966). Factors determining the maximal rate of organic anion secretion by the liver and further evidence on the hepatic site of action of the hormone secretin. *J. Physiol.* **186**, 424-438.

493. O'Máille, E. R. L., Richards, T. G. & Short, A. H. (1967). The influence of conjugation of cholic acid on its uptake and secretion: hepatic extraction of taurocholate and cholate in the dog. *J. Physiol.* **189**, 337-350.

494. Osborne, E. C., Wootton, I. D. P., Da Silva, L. C. & Sherlock, S. (1959). Serum bile-acid-levels in liver disease. *Lancet* **2**, 1049-1053.

495. Ostrow, J. D. (1969). Absorption by the gallbladder of bile salts, sulfobromophthalein and iodipamide. *J. Lab. clin. Med.* **74**, 482-494.

496. Osuga, T. & Portman, O. W. (1971). Experimental formation of gallstones in the squirrel monkey. *Proc. Soc. exp. Biol. Med.* **136**, 722-726.

497. Overholt, B. F. & Pollard, H. M. (1968). Acid diffusion into the human gastric mucosa. *Gastroenterology* **54**, 182-189.

498. Painter, N. S. & Burkitt, D. P. (1971). Diverticular disease of the colon: a deficiency disease of Western civilisation. *Br. med. J.* **2**, 450-454.

499. Palmer, R. H. (1967). The formation of bile acid sulfates: a new pathway of bile acid metabolism in humans. *Proc. natn. Acad. Sci. U.S.A.* **58**, 1047-1050.

500. Palmer, R. H. (1969). Toxic effects of lithocholic acid and related 5β-H steroids. In *Bile Salt Metabolism.* ed. Schiff, L., Carey, J. B. & Dietschy, J. M., pp. 184-204. Springfield: Thomas.

501. Palmer, R. H., Glickman, P. B. & Kappas, A. (1962). Pyrogenic and inflammatory properties of certain bile acids in man. *J. clin. Invest.* **41**, 1573-1577.

502. Palmer, R. H. & Hruban, Z. (1966). Production of bile duct hyperplasia and gallstones by lithocholic acid. *J. clin. Invest.* **45**, 1255-1267.

503. Panveliwalla, D., Lewis, B., Wootton, I. D. P. & Tabaqchali, S. (1970). Determination of individual bile acids in biological fluids by thin-layer chromatography and fluorimetry. *J. clin. Path.* **23**, 309-314.

504. Parkinson, T. M. (1967). Hypolipidemic effects of orally administered dextran and cellulose anion exchangers in cockerels and dogs. *J. Lipid Res.* **8**, 24-29.

505. Paulley, J. W. (1969). The jejunal mucosa in malabsorptive states with high bacterial counts. In *Malabsorption*, ed. Girdwood, R. H. & Smith, A. N. (Pfizer Monograph), pp. 171-176. University of Edinburgh Press.

506. Percy-Robb, I. W. & Boyd, G. S. (1968). The enterohepatic circulation of bile salts. In *The Liver*, ed. Read, A. E., pp. 11-15. London: Butterworths.

507. Percy-Robb, I. W., Brunton, W. A. T., Jalan, K. N., McManus, J. P. A., Gould, J. C. & Sircus, W. (1969). The relationship between the bacterial content of ileal effluent and the metabolism of bile salts in patients with ileostomies. *Gut* **10**, 1049-1050 (abstract).

508. Percy-Robb, I. W., Jalan, K. N., McManus, J. P. A. & Sircus, W. (1971). Effect of ileal resection on bile salt metabolism in patients with ileostomy following proctocolectomy. *Clin. Sci.* **41**, 371-382.

509. Pfaff, F. & Balch, A. W. (1897). An experimental investigation of some of the conditions influencing the secretion and composition of human bile. *J. exp. Med.* **2**, 49-105.

510. Philippon, F. & Kern, F. (1968). Fatty acid absorption in the absence of bile salts: morphological and biochemical observations. *Gastroenterology* **54**, 1299 (abstract).

511. Philippon, F. & Kern, F. (1969). Effects of bile depletion on absorption, esterification and transport of long chain fatty acid. *Gastroenterology* **56**, 1260 (abstract).

512. Playoust, M. R. & Isselbacher, K. J. (1964). Studies on the transport and metabolism of conjugated bile salts by intestinal mucosa. *J. clin. Invest.* **43**, 467-476.

513. Playoust, M. R., Lack, L. & Weiner, I. M. (1965). Effect of intestinal resection on bile salt absorption in dogs. *Am. J. Physiol.* **208**, 363-369.

514. Poley, J. R., Dower, J. C., Owen, C. A. & Stickler, G. B. (1964). Bile acids in infants and children. *J. Lab. clin. Med.* **63**, 838-846.

515. Poley, J. R. & Hofmann, A. F. (1968). Diarrhea following ileal resection: pathogenesis and treatment. *J. clin. Invest.* **47**, 79A-80A (abstract).

516. Poley, J. R., Smith, J. D., Thompson, J. B. & Seely, J. R. (1971).

The influence of growth hormone on intestinal micellar bile acids during digestion in man. *Gastroenterology* **60**, 707 (abstract).

517. Pomare, E. & Heaton, K. W. (1971). Unpublished studies.

518. Pope, J. L., Parkinson, T. M. & Olson, J. A. (1966). Action of bile salts on the metabolism and transport of water-soluble nutrients by perfused rat jejunum *in vitro*. *Biochim. biophys. Acta* **130**, 218-232.

519. Porter, H. P., Saunders, D. R., Brunser, O., Tytgat, G. N. & Rubin, C. E. (1970). Fat absorption in bile fistula man: a clue to the pathway of normal fatty acid absorption. *Gastroenterology* **58**, 984 (abstract).

520. Porter, H. P., Saunders, D. R., Tytgat, G., Brunser, O. & Rubin, C. E. (1971). Fat absorption in bile fistula man. A morphological and biochemical study. *Gastroenterology* **60**, 1008-1019.

521. Portman, O. W. (1960). Nutritional influences on the metabolism of bile acids. *Am. J. clin. Nutr.* **8**, 462-470.

522. Portman, O. W. (1962). Importance of diet, species and intestinal flora in bile acid metabolism. *Fedn Proc.* **21**, 896-902.

523. Portman, O. W., Lawry, E. Y. & Bruno, D. (1956). Effect of dietary carbohydrate on experimentally induced hypercholesteremia and hyperbetalipoproteinemia in rats. *Proc. Soc. exp. Biol. Med.* **91**, 321-323.

524. Portman, O. W., Mann, G. V. & Wysocki, A. P. (1955). Bile acid excretion by the rat: nutritional effects. *Archs Biochem. Biophys.* **59**, 224-232.

525. Portman, O. W. & Murphy, P. (1958). Excretion of bile acids and β-hydroxysterols by rats. *Archs Biochem. Biophys.* **76**, 367-376.

526. Portman, O. W. & Shah, S. (1962). determination of concentrations of bile acids in peripheral, portal and hepatic blood in Cebus monkeys. *Archs Biochem. Biophys.* **96**, 516-523.

527. Quintão, E., Grundy, S. M. & Ahrens, E. H. (1971). Effects of dietary cholesterol on the regulation of total body cholesterol in man. *J. Lipid Res.* **12**, 233-247.

528. Rautureau, M., Chevrel, B. & Caroli, J. (1967). Les acides biliaires sanguins en hépatologie. VI. Conclusions d'une étude portant sur 195 malades et bibliographie. *Rev. med. chir. Mal. Foie* **42**, 232-236.

529. Redinger, R. N., Herman, A. H. & Small, D. M. (1971). Effect of diet on bile composition in the Rhesus monkey. *Gastroenterology* **60**, 198 (abstract).

530. Redinger, R. N. & Small, D. M. (1971). The effect of phenobarbital on bile salt metabolism and cholesterol secretion in the primate. *J. clin. Invest.* **50**, 76A (abstract).

531. Rhodes, J. (1972). The aetiology of gastric ulcer. *Gastroenterology*, in press.

532. Rhodes, J., Barnardo, D. E., Phillips, S. F., Rovelstad, R. A. & Hofmann, A. F. (1969). Increased reflux of bile into the stomach in patients with gastric ulcer. *Gastroenterology* **57**, 241-252.

533. Riccardi, B. A. & Fahrenbach, M. J. (1966). Effect of guar gum and pectin N.F. on serum and liver lipids of cholesterol-fed rats. *Proc. Soc. exp. Biol. Med.* **124**, 749-752.

534. Robinson, H. J., Kelley, K. L. & Lehman, E. G. (1964). Effect of cholestyramine, a bile acid binding polymer, on vitamin K_1 absorption in dogs. *Proc. Soc. exp. Biol. Med.* **115**, 112-115.

535. Roepke, R. R. & Mason, H. L. (1940). Micelle formation in aqueous solutions of bile salts. *J. biol. Chem.* **133**, 103-108.

536. Rogers, A. I., Bachorik, P. S. & Johnson, M. (1971). The role of bile salts in fatty acid assimilation by rat small intestine. *Gastroenterology* **60**, 797 (abstract).

537. Rosenberg, I. H. (1969). Influence of intestinal bacteria on bile acid metabolism and fat absorption. *Am. J. clin. Nutr.* **22**, 284-291.

538. Rosenberg, I. H., Hardison, W. G. & Bull, D. M. (1967). Abnormal bile-salt patterns and intestinal bacterial overgrowth associated with malabsorption. *New Engl. J. Med.* **276**, 1391-1397.

539. Rosenfeld, R. S. & Hellman, L. (1962). Excretion of steroid acids in man. *Archs Biochem. Biophys.* **97**, 406-410.

540. Rosenheim, O. & King, H. (1932). The ring system of sterols and bile acids. Part II. *Chem. Ind.* **10**, 954-956.

541. Rowe, G. G. (1967). Control of tenesmus and diarrhea by cholestyramine administration. *Gastroenterology* **53**, 1006.

542. Rubulis, A., Rubert, M. & Faloon, W. W. (1970). Cholesterol lowering, fecal bile acid, and sterol changes during neomycin and colchicine. *Am. J. clin. Nutr.* **23**, 1251-1259.

543. Rudman, D. & Kendall, F. E. (1957). Bile acid content of human serum. I. Serum bile acids in patients with hepatic disease. *J. clin. Invest.* **36**, 530-537.

544. Sallee, V. L. & Dietschy, J. M. (1971). The role of bile acid micelles in absorption of fatty acids across the intestinal brush border. *J. clin. Invest.* **50**, 80A-81A (abstract).

545. Salmon, P. R., Low-Beer, T. S. & Heaton, K. W. (1971). Unpublished observations.

546. Salmon, P. R., McCarthy, C. F. & Read, A. E. (1969). An isotope technique for measuring lactose absorption. *Gut* **10**, 685-689.

547. Sampliner, R. E., Bennett, P. H., Comess, L. J., Rose, F. A. & Burch, T. A. (1970). Gallbladder disease in Pima Indians. Demonstration of high prevalence and early onset by cholecystography. *New Engl. J. Med.* **283**, 1358-1364.

548. Samuel, P., Saypol, G. M., Meilman, E., Mosbach, E. H. & Chafizadeh, M. (1968). Absorption of bile acids from the large bowel in man. *J. clin. Invest.* **47**, 2070-2078.

549. Sandberg, D. H., Sjövall, J., Sjövall, K. & Turner, D. A. (1965). Measurement of human serum bile acids by gas-liquid chromatography. *J. Lipid Res.* **6**, 182-192.

550. Sarles, H., Chabert, C., Pommeau, Y., Save, E., Mouret, H. & Gérolami, A. (1969). Diet and cholesterol gallstones. A study of 101 patients with cholelithiasis compared to 101 matched controls. *Am. J. dig. Dis.* **14**, 531-537.

551. Sarles, H., Crotte, C., Gérolami, A., Mule, A., Domingo, N. & Hauton, J. (1970). Influence of cholestyramine, bile salt, and cholesterol feeding on the lipid composition of hepatic bile in man. *Scand. J. Gastroent.* **5**, 603-608.

552. Sarles, H., Hauton, J., Lafont, H., Teissier, N., Planche, N.-E. & Gérolami, A. (1968). Role de l'alimentation sur la concentration du cholestérol biliaire chez l'homme lithiasique et non-lithiasique. *Clin. chim. Acta* **19**, 147-155.

553. Sarles, H., Hauton, J., Planche, N. E., Lafont, H. & Gérolami, A. (1970). Diet, cholesterol gallstones, and composition of the bile. *Am. J. dig. Dis.* **15**, 251-260.

554. Saunders, D. R. (1970). Insignificance of the enterobiliary circulation of lecithin in man. *Gastroenterology* **59**, 848-852.

555. Schachter, D., Finkelstein, J. D. & Kowarski, S. (1964). Metabolism of vitamin D. I. Preparation of radioactive vitamin D and its intestinal absorption in the rat. *J. clin. Invest.* **43**, 787-796.

556. Schaffner, F. (1964). Cholestyramine, a boon to some who itch. *Gastroenterology* **46**, 67-70.

557. Schaffner, F. & Popper, H. (1969). Cholestasis is the result of hypoactive hypertrophic smooth endoplasmic reticulum in the hepatocyte. *Lancet* **2**, 355-359.

558. Schapiro, R. H., Heizer, W. D., Goldfinger, S. E. & Aserkoff, B. R. (1970). Cholestyramine responsive idiopathic diarrhea. *Gastroenterology* **58**, 993 (abstract).

559. Schellbach, R. (1851). Ueber die Funktion der Galle. *Justus Leibigs Annln Chem.* **79**, 290-313.

560. Schersten, T. (1967). The synthesis of cholic acid conjugates in human liver. *Acta chir. scand. Supp.* 373.

561. Schiff, E. R. & Dietschy, J. M. (1968). Comparative kinetics of active transport of bile acid analogues. *J. clin. Invest.* **47**, 87A (abstract).

562. Schiff, E. R. & Dietschy, J. M. (1969). Current concepts of bile acid absorption. *Am. J. clin. Nutr.* **22**, 273-278.

563. Schiff, M. (1870). Bericht über einige Versuchsreihen. I. Gallenbildung, abhängig der Aufsaugung der Gallenstoffe. *Pflügers Arch. ges. Physiol.* **3**, 598-613.

564. Schiff, M. (1892). Cited by Sobotka (1937).

565. Schmidt, C. R., Beazell, J. M., Berman, A. L., Ivy, A. C. & Atkinson, A. J. (1939). Studies on the secretion of bile. *Am. J. Physiol.* **126**, 120-135.

566. Schmidt, H. & Creutzfeldt, W. (1969). The possible role of phospholipase A in the pathogenesis of acute pancreatitis. *Scand. J. Gastroent.* **4**, 39-48.

567. Schoenfield, L. J. (1969). The relationship of bile acids to pruritus in hepatobiliary disease. In *Bile Salt Metabolism*, ed. Schiff, L., Carey, J. B. & Dietschy, J. M., pp. 257-265. Springfield: Thomas.

568. Schoenfield, L. J. & Foulk, W. T. (1964). Studies of sulfobromophthalein sodium (BSP) metabolism in man. II. The effect of artificially induced fever, norethandrolone (Nilevar), and iopanoic acid (Telepaque). *J. clin. Invest.* **43**, 1419-1423.

569. Schoenfield, L. J. & Sjövall, J. (1966). Bile acids and cholesterol in guinea pigs with induced gallstones. *Am. J. Physiol.* **211**, 1069-1074.

570. Schoenfield, L. J., Sjövall, J. & Perman, E. (1967). Bile acids on the skin of patients with pruritic hepatobiliary disease. *Nature, Lond.* **213**, 93-94.

571. Schoenfield, L. J., Sjövall, J. & Sjövall, K. (1966). Bile acid composition of gallstones from man. *J. Lab. clin. Med.* **68**, 186-194.

572. Schultz, S. G. & Strecker, C. K. (1971). Cholesterol and bile salt fluxes across brush border of rat jejunum. *Am. J. Physiol.* **220**, 59-65.

573. Schüpbach, A. (1907). Cited by Hertz, A. F. (1909). *Constipation and Allied Intestinal Disorders*. London: Frowde.

574. Schwann, T. (1844). Cited by Garrison, F. H. (1929). *History of Medicine*, 4th edn, p. 456. Philadelphia: Saunders.

575. Scott, H. W., Stephenson, S. E., Hayes, C. W. & Younger, R. K. (1967). Effects of bypass of the distal fourth of small intestine on experimental hypercholesterolemia and atherosclerosis in Rhesus monkeys. *Surgery, Gynec. Obstet.* **125**, 3-12.

576. Scott, H. W., Stephenson, S. E., Younger, R., Carlisle, B. B. & Turney, S. W. (1966). Prevention of experimental atherosclerosis by ileal bypass. *Ann. Surg.* **163**, 795-807.

577. Sharp, H. L., Carey, J. B., White, J. G. & Krivit, W. (1967). Cholestyramine therapy in patients with a paucity of intrahepatic bile ducts. *J. Pediat.* **71**, 723-736.

578. Shefer, S., Hauser, S. Bekersky, I. & Mosbach, E. H. (1969). Feedback regulation of bile acid biosynthesis in the rat. *J. Lipid Res.* **10**, 646-655.

579. Shefer, S., Hauser, S., Bekersky, I. & Mosbach, E. H. (1970). Biochemical site of regulation of bile acid biosynthesis in the rat. *J. Lipid Res.* **11**, 404-411.

580. Sherlock, S. (1968). *Diseases of the Liver and Biliary System*. 4th edn, p. 287. Oxford: Blackwell.

581. Sherr, H. P., Newman, A., Sasaki, Y., Banwell, J. G. & Hendrix, T. R. (1971). Detection of bacterial deconjugation of bile salts by a convenient breath analysis technique. *Gastroenterology* **60**, 801 (abstract).

582. Shimada, K., Bricknell, K. S. & Finegold, S. M. (1969). Deconjugation of bile acids by intestinal bacteria: review of literature and additional studies. *J. inf. Dis.* **119**, 273-281.

583. Shiner, M. (1969). Effect of bile acids on the small intestinal mucosa in man and rats; a light and electron microscope study. In *Bile Salt Metabolism*, ed. Schiff, L., Carey, J. B. & Dietschy, J. M., pp. 41-55. Springfield: Thomas.

584. Shurpalekar, K. S., Doraiswamy, T. R., Sundaravalli, O. E. & Narayana Rao, M. (1971). Effect of inclusion of cellulose in an 'atherogenic' diet on the blood lipids of children. *Nature, Lond.* **232**, 554-555.

585. Shuster, F., Spoto, R. C. & Jacobs, M. N. (1970). Cholestyramine and polysorbate-80 in the treatment of cholerheic enteropathy. *Am. J. dig. Dis.* **15**, 353-358.

586. Siegel, R. E. (1968). *Galen's System of Physiology and Medicine*, p. 216. Basel: Karger.

587. Simmonds, W. J. (1969). Effect of bile salts on the rate of fat absorption. *Am. J. clin. Nutr.* **22**, 266-272.

588. Simmonds, W. J., Hofmann, A. F. & Theodor, E. (1967). Absorption of cholesterol from a micellar solution: intestinal perfusion studies in man. *J. clin. Invest.* **46**, 874-890.

589. Simmonds, W. J., Redgrave, T. G. & Willix, R. L. S. (1968). Absorption of oleic and palmitic acids from emulsions and micellar solutions. *J. clin. Invest.* **47**, 1015-1025.

590. Singleton, A. O., Redmond, D. C. & McMurray, J. E. (1964). Ileocecal resection and small bowel transit and absorption. *Ann. Surg.* **159**, 690-693.

591. Siperstein, M. D., Chaikoff, I. L. & Reinhardt, W. O. (1952). C^{14}-cholesterol. V. Obligatory function of bile in intestinal absorption of cholesterol. *J. biol. Chem.* **198**, 111-114.

592. Siperstein, M. D., Nichols, C. W. & Chaikoff, I. L. (1953). Effects of ferric chloride and bile on plasma cholesterol and atherosclerosis in the cholesterol-fed bird. *Science* **117**, 386-389.

593. Sjövall, J. (1955). Quantitative determination of bile acids on paper chromatograms. *Ark. Kemi* **8**, 317-324.

594. Sjövall, J. (1959a). On the concentration of bile acids in the human intestine during absorption. *Acta physiol. scand.* **46**, 339-345.

595. Sjövall, J. (1959b). Dietary glycine and taurine on bile acid conjugation in man. *Proc. Soc. exp. Biol. Med.* **100**, 676-678.

596. Sjövall, J. (1960). Bile acids in man under normal and pathological conditions. *Clin. chim. Acta* **5**, 33-41.

597. Sjövall, J. (1964). Separation and determination of bile acids. In *Methods of Biochemical Analysis,* Vol. 12, ed. Glick, D., pp. 97-141. New York: Interscience.

598. Sjövall, J. (1969). Use of gas chromatography–mass spectrometry in the study of bile acid metabolism. In *Bile Salt Metabolism,* ed. Schiff, L., Carey, J. B. & Dietschy, J. M., pp. 205-222. Springfield: Thomas.

599. Sjövall, J. & Åkesson, I. (1955). Intestinal absorption of taurocholic acid in the rat. *Acta physiol. scand.* **34**, 278-286.

600. Sjövall, K. & Sjövall, J. (1966). Serum bile acid levels in pregnancy with pruritus. *Clin. chim. Acta* **13**, 207-211.

601. Skillman, J. Gould, S. A., Chung, R. S. K. & Silen, W. (1970). The gastric mucosal barrier: clinical and experimental studies in critically ill and normal man and in the rabbit. *Ann. Surg.* **172**, 564-584.

602. Small, D. M. (1968). Gallstones. *New Engl. J. Med.* **279**, 588-593.
603. Small, D. M. (1970a). The formation of gallstones. *Adv. internal Med.* **16**, 243-264.
604. Small, D. M. (1970b). Surface and bulk interactions of lipids and water with a classification of biologically active lipids based on these interactions. *Fedn Proc.* **29**, 1320-1326.
605. Small, D. M. (1971). Prestone gallstone disease—is therapy safe? *New Engl. J. Med.* **284**, 214-216.
606. Small, D. M. & Admirand, W. H. (1969). Solubility of bile salts. *Nature, Lond.* **221**, 265-267.
607. Smali, D. M., Bourges, M. & Dervichian, D. G. (1966). Ternary and quaternary aqueous systems containing bile salt, lecithin and cholesterol. *Nature, Lond.* **211**, 816-818.
608. Small, D. M. & Rapo, S. (1970). Source of abnormal bile in patients with cholesterol gallstones. *New Engl. J. Med.* **283**, 53-57.
609. Small, N. C. & Dietschy, J. M. (1968). Characterisation of the monomer and micelle components of the passive diffusion process of bile acids across the small intestine of the rat. *Gastroenterology* **54**, 1272 (abstract).
610. Smith, H. P. & Whipple, G. H. (1928). Bile salt metabolism. II. Influence of meat and meat extractives, liver and kidney, egg yolk and yeast in the diet. *J. biol. Chem.* **80**, 671-684.
610a. Smith, L. H., Fromm, H. & Hofmann, A. F. (1972). Acquired hyperoxaluria, nephrolithiasis and intestinal disease: description of a new syndrome. *New Engl. J. Med.* In the press.
611. Smyth, F. S. & Whipple, G. H. (1924). Bile salt metabolism. I. Influence of chloroform and phosphorus on bile fistula dogs. *J. biol. Chem.* **59**, 623-636.
612. Snog-Kjaer, A., Prange, I., Christensen, F. & Dam, H. (1963). Alimentary production of gallstones in hamsters. 12. Studies with rice starch diets with and without antibiotics. *Z. Ernährungsw.* **4**, 14-25.
613. Sobotka, H. (1937). *Physiological Chemistry of the Bile.* London: Baillière, Tindall & Cox.
614. Sobotka, H. (1938). *The Chemistry of the Sterids.* London: Baillière, Tindall & Cox.
615. Södal, G., Gjertsen, K. T. & Schrumpf, A. (1970). Surgical treatment of hypercholesterolemia. *Acta chir. scand.* **136**, 671-674.
616. Southgate, D. A. T. & Durnin, J. V. G. A. (1970). Calorie conversion factors. An experimental reassessment of the

factors used in the calculation of the energy value of human diets. *Br. J. Nutr.* **24**, 517-535.

617. Sperber, I. (1959). Secretion of organic anions in the formation of urine and bile. *Pharmac. Rev.* **11**, 109-134.

618. Sperber, I. (1965). Biliary secretion of organic anions and its influence on bile flow. In *The Biliary System,* ed. Taylor, W., pp. 457-467. Oxford: Blackwell.

619. Stacey, M. & Webb, M. (1947). Studies on the antibacterial properties of the bile acids and some compounds derived from cholanic acid. *Proc. roy. Soc. B.* **134**, 523-537.

620. Stahlgren, L. H., Umana, G., Roy, R. & Donnelly, J. (1962). A study of intestinal absorption in dogs following massive small intestinal resection and insertion of an antiperistaltic segment. *Ann. Surg.* **156**, 483-491.

621. Standaert, L. O. (1967). Experimental gallstone formation in the animal. *Proc. 3rd World Congress Gastroenterology, Tokyo 1966.* Vol. 4, pp. 101-108. Basel: Karger.

622. Stanley, M. M. & Nemchausky, B. (1967). Fecal C^{14}-bile acid excretion in normal subjects and patients with steroid-wasting syndromes secondary to ileal dysfunction. *J. Lab. clin. Med.* **70**, 627-639.

623. Stathers, G. M. (1966). Porphyrin-binding effect of cholestyramine. Results of *in-vitro* and *in-vivo* studies. *Lancet* **2**, 780-783.

624. Stiehl, A., Admirand, W. H. & Thaler, M. M. (1971). Effects of phenobarbital on intrahepatic and extrahepatic cholestasis. *Gastroenterology* **60**, 183 (abstract).

625. Stiehl, A. Wollenweber, J. & Wagener, H. (1969). Die dünnschichtchromatographische Trennung der freien Gallensäuren im Durchlaufverfahren und ihre Isolierung mit einem modifizierten Leitchromatogramm. *J. Chromatog.* **43**, 278-281.

626. Stout, R. W. (1970). Development of vascular lesions in insulin treated animals fed a normal diet. *Br. med. J.* **3**, 685-687.

627. Stout, R. W. & Vallance-Owen, J. W. (1969). Insulin and atheroma. *Lancet* **1**, 1078-1080.

628. Strand, O. (1962). Influence of propylthiouracil and D- and L-triiodothyronine on excretion of bile acids in bile fistula rats. *Proc. Soc. exp. Biol. Med.* **109**, 668-672.

629. Strand, O. (1963). Effects of D- and L-triiodothyronine and of propylthiouracil on the production of bile acids in the rat. *J. Lipid Res.* **4**, 305-311.

630. Strecker, A. (1848). Untersuchung der Ochsengalle. *Justus Liebigs Annln Chem.* **65**, 1-37.

631. Sullivan, M. F. (1965). Bile salt absorption in the irradiated rat. *Am. J. Physiol.* **209**, 158-164.

632. Sundaravalli, O. E., Shurpalekar, K. S. & Narayana Rao, M. N. (1971). Effects of dietary cellulose supplements on the body composition and cholesterol metabolism of albino rats. *J. Agr. Food Chem.* **19**, 116-118.

633. Sutor, D. J. & Wooley, S. E. (1971). A statistical survey of the composition of gallstones in eight countries. *Gut* **12**, 55-64.

634. Swan, D. C., Davidson, P. & Albrink, M. J. (1966). Effect of simple and complex carbohydrates on plasma non-esterified fatty acids, plasma-sugar, and plasma-insulin during oral carbohydrate tolerance tests. *Lancet* **1**, 60-63.

635. Swell, L. (1968). *Gas Chromatography*, pp. 97-109. New York: Grune & Stratton.

636. Swell, L., Bell, C. C. & Entenman, C. (1968). Bile acids and lipid metabolism. III. Influence of bile acids on phospholipids in liver and bile of the isolated perfused dog liver. *Biochim. biophys. Acta* **164**, 278-284.

637. Swell, L., Bell, C. C. & Vlahcevic, Z. R. (1971). Relationship of bile acid pool size to the formation of lithogenic bile in man. *Gastroenterology* **60**, 723 (abstract).

638. Swell, L., Entenman, C., Leong, G. F. & Holloway, R. J. (1968). Bile acids and lipid metabolism. IV. Influence of bile acids on biliary and liver organelle phospholipids and cholesterol. *Am. J. Physiol.* **215**, 1390-1396.

639. Switz, D. M., Hislop, I. G. & Hofmann, A. F. (1970). Factors influencing the absorption of bile acids by the human jejunum. *Gastroenterology* **58**, 999 (abstract).

640. Sylvén, C. & Nordström, C. (1970). The site of absorption of cholesterol and sitosterol in the rat small intestine. *Scand. J. Gastroent.* **5**, 57-63.

641. Szalkowski, C. R. & Mader, W. J. (1952). Colorimetric determination of desoxycholic acid in ox bile. *Anal. Chem.* **24**, 1602-1604.

642. Tabaqchali, S. (1970). The pathophysiological role of small intestinal bacterial flora. *Scand. J. Gastroent. Supp.* **6**, 139-163.

643. Tabaqchali, S. & Booth, C. C. (1966). Jejunal bacteriology and bile-salt metabolism in patients with intestinal malabsorption. *Lancet* **2**, 12-15.

644. Tabaqchali, S. & Booth, C. C. (1970). Bacteria and the small intestine. In *Modern Trends in Gastroenterology—4.* Ed. Card, W. I. & Creamer, B., pp. 143-179. London: Butterworths.

645. Tabaqchali, S., Hatzioannou, J. & Booth, C. C. (1968). Bile-salt deconjugation and steatorrhoea in patients with the stagnant loop syndrome. *Lancet* 2, 12-16.

646. Talalay, P. (1960). Enzymic analysis of steroid hormones. In *Methods of Biochemical Analysis,* Vol. 8, ed. Blick, D., pp. 119-143. New York: Interscience.

647. Tamesue, N. & Juniper, K. (1967). Concentrations of bile salts at the critical micellar concentration of human gall bladder bile. *Gastroenterology* 52, 473-479.

648. Tappeiner, H. (1878). Ueber die Aufsaugung der Gallensäuren Alkalien in Dünndarme. *Sber. Akad. Wiss. Wien. Abt. III,* 77, 281-304.

649. Tennent, D. M., Hashim, S. A. & van Itallie, T. B. (1962). Bile-acid sequestrants and lipid metabolism. *Fedn Proc.* 21, supp. 11, 77-80.

650. Tennent, D. M., Siegel, H., Zanetti, M. E., Kuron, G. W., Ott, W. H. & Wolf, F. J. (1960). Plasma cholesterol lowering action of bile acid binding polymers in experimental animals. *J. Lipid Res.* 1, 469-473.

651. Tepperman, J., Caldwell, F. T. & Tepperman, H. M. (1964). Induction of gallstones in mice by feeding a cholesterol-cholic acid containing diet. *Am. J. Physiol.* 206, 628-634.

653. Theodor, E., Spritz, N. & Sleisenger, M. H. (1968). Metabolism of intravenously injected isotopic cholic acid in viral hepatitis. *Gastroenterology* 55, 183-190.

654. Thiffault, C., Bélanger, M. & Pouliot, M. (1970). Traitement de l'hyperlipoprotéinémie essentielle de type II par un nouvel agent thérapeutique, la celluline. *Can. med. Ass. J.* 103, 165-166.

655. Thistle, J. L. & Schoenfield, L. J. (1968). Lecithin, and cholesterol in repeated human duodenal biliary drainage; effect of lecithin feeding. *Clin. Res.* 16, 450 (abstract).

656. Thistle, J. L. & Schoenfield, L. J. (1971). Lithogenic bile among young Indian women. Lithogenic potential decreased with chenodeoxycholic acid. *New Engl. J. Med.* 284, 177-181.

657. Thomas, P. J., Hsia, S. L., Matschiner, J. T., Doisy, E. A., Elliott, W. H., Thayer, S. A. & Doisy, E. A. (1964). Bile acids. XIX. Metabolism of lithocholic acid-24-^{14}C in the rat. *J. biol. Chem.* 239, 102-105.

658. Thompson, G. R., Barrowman, J., Gutierrez, L. & Dowling, R. H. (1971). Action of neomycin on the intraluminal phase of lipid absorption. *J. clin. Invest.* **50**, 319-323.

659. Thompson, G. R., Ockner, R. K. & Isselbacher, K. J. (1969). Effect of mixed micellar lipid on the absorption of cholesterol and vitamin D_3 into lymph. *J. clin. Invest.* **48**, 87-95.

660. Thompson, W. G. & Thompson, G. R. (1969). Effect of cholestyramine on the absorption of vitamin D_3 and calcium. *Gut* **10**, 717-722.

661. Thornton, A. G., Vahouny, G. V. & Treadwell, C. R. (1968). Absorption of lipids from mixed micellar solutions. *Proc. Soc. exp. biol. Med.* **127**, 629-632.

662. Thureborn, E. (1962). Human hepatic bile. Composition changes due to altered enterohepatic circulation. *Acta chir. scand. Supp.* **303**.

663. Tidball, C. S. (1964). Intestinal and hepatic transport of cholate and organic dyes. *Am. J. Physiol.* **206**, 239-242.

664. Tompkins, R. K., Burke, L. G., Zollinger, R. M. & Cornwell, D. G. (1970). Relationship of biliary phospholipid and cholesterol concentrations to the occurrence and dissolution of human gallstones. *Ann. Surg.* **172**, 936-945.

665. Treadwell, C. R. & Vahouny, G. V. (1968). Cholesterol absorption. In *Handbook of Physiology*, section 6: Alimentary canal, Vol. 3: Intestinal absorption, ed. Code, C. F., pp. 1407-1438. Washington: American Physiological Society.

666. Trowell, H. C. (1972). Dietary fibre and coronary heart disease. *Rev. eur. d'Etudes clin. biol.* (in press).

667. Tucker, P., Lanz, H. & Senior, J. (1970). Intracellular role of bile salts in release into lymph of lipids synthesised in the intestinal mucosa. *Fedn Proc.* **29**, 844 (abstract).

668. Turnberg, L. A. & Anthony-Mote, A. (1969). The quantitative determination of bile salts in bile using thin-layer chromatography and 3α-hydroxysteroid dehydrogenase. *Clin. chim. Acta* **24**, 253-259.

669. Turnberg, L. A. & Grahame, G. (1970). Bile salt secretion in cirrhosis of the liver. *Gut* **11**, 126-133.

670. Turner, M. D., Bevan, G., Engert, R., Klipstein, F. & Maldonado, N. (1970). Bile salt metabolism in tropical sprue. *Gastroenterology* **58**, 1002 (abstract).

671. Usui, T. (1963). Thin-layer chromatography of bile acids with special reference to separation of keto bile acids. *J. Biochem.* **54**, 283-286.

672. van Belle, H. (1965). *Cholesterol, Bile Acids and Atherosclerosis.* Amsterdam: North Holland Publishing Company.

673. van Deest, B. W., Fordtran, J. S., Morawski, S. G. & Wilson, J. D. (1968). Bile salt and micellar fat concentration in proximal small bowel contents of ileectomy patients. *J. clin. Invest.* **47**, 1314-1324.

674. van der Linden, W. (1971). Bile acid patterns of patients with and without gallstones. *Gastroenterology* **60**, 1144-1145.

675. van der Linden, W. & Nakayama, F. (1969). Change of bile composition in man after administration of cholestyramine (a gallstone dissolving agent in hamsters). *Acta chir. scand.* **135**, 433-438.

676. van Itallie, T. B. & Hashim, S. A. (1963). Clinical and experimental aspects of bile acid metabolism. *Med. Clin. N. Amer.* **47**, 629-648.

677. van Itallie, T. B., Hashim, S. A., Crampton, R. S. & Tennent, D. M. (1961). The treatment of pruritus and hypercholesteremia of primary biliary cirrhosis with cholestyramine. *New Engl. J. Med.* **265**, 469-474.

678. Verzár, F. & McDougall, E. J. (1936). *Absorption from the Intestine.* London: Longmans.

679. Vlahcevic, Z. R., Bell, C. C., Buhac, I., Farrar, J. T. & Swell, L. (1970). Diminished bile acid pool size in patients with gallstones. *Gastroenterology* **59**, 165-173.

680. Vlahcevic, Z. R., Bell, C. C., Gregory, D. H., Buker, G., Juttijudata, P. & Swell, L. (1972). Relationship of bile acid pool size to the formation of lithogenic bile in female Indians of the Southwest. *Gastroenterology* **62**, 73-83.

681. Vlahcevic, Z. R., Bell, C. C. & Swell, L. (1970). Significance of the liver in the production of lithogenic bile in man. *Gastroenterology* **59**, 62-69.

682. Vlahcevic, Z. R., Buhac, I., Bell, C. C. & Swell, L. (1970). Abnormal metabolism of secondary bile acids in patients with cirrhosis. *Gut* **11**, 420-422.

683. Vlahcevic, Z. R., Buhac, I., Farrar, J. T., Bell, C. C. & Swell, L. (1971). Bile acid metabolism in patients with cirrhosis. I. Kinetic aspects of cholic acid metabolism. *Gastroenterology* **60**, 491-498.

684. Vlahcevic, Z. R., Miller, J. R., Farrar, J. T. & Swell, L. (1971). Kinetics and pool size of primary bile acids in man. *Gastroenterology* **61**, 85-90.

685. Wachtel, N., Emerman, S. & Javitt, N. B. (1968). Metabolism of

cholest-5-ene-3β, 26-diol in the rat and hamster. *J. biol. Chem.* **243**, 5207-5212.

686. Watanabe, N., Gimbel, N. S. & Johnston, C. G. (1962). Effect of polyunsaturated and saturated fatty acids on the cholesterol holding capacity of human bile. *Archs Surg., Chicago* **85**, 136-141.

687. Webling, D. D'a. (1966). The site of absorption of taurocholate in chicks, using polyethylene glycol as a reference substance. *Aust. J. exp. Biol. med. Sci.* **44**, 101-104.

688. Webling, D. D'A. & Holdsworth, E. S. (1966a). Bile salts and calcium absorption. *Biochem. J.* **100**, 652-660.

689. Webling, D. D'A. & Holdsworth, E. S. (1966b). Bile and the absorption of strontium and iron. *Biochem. J.* **100**, 661-663.

690. Weiner, I. M. & Lack, L. (1962). Absorption of bile salts from the small intestine *in vivo. Am. J. Physiol.* **202**, 155-157.

691. Weiner, I. M. & Lack, L. (1968). Bile salt absorption; enterohepatic circulation. In *Handbook of Physiology,* Section 6: Alimentary Canal, Vol. III: Intestinal Absorption, ed. Code, C. F., pp. 1439-1455. Washington: American Physiological Society.

692. Weis, H. J. & Dietschy, J. M. (1969). Failure of bile acids to control hepatic cholesterogenesis: evidence for endogenous cholesterol feedback. *J. clin. Invest.* **48**, 2398-2408.

693. Weiss, A. (1884). Ce que devient la bile dans le canal digestif. *Bull. Soc. imp. des Nat. de Moscou* **59**, 22-32.

694. Weiss, J. B. & Holt, P. R. (1971). Controlling factors during intestinal fat absorption in man. *J. clin. Invest.* **50**, 97A (abstract).

695. Wheeler, H. O. (1965). Inorganic ions in bile. In *The Biliary System,* ed. Taylor, W., pp. 481-491. Oxford: Blackwell.

696. Wheeler, H. O. (1969). Secretion of bile. In *Diseases of the Liver,* ed. Schiff, L., 3rd edition, pp. 84-102. Philadelphia: Lippincott.

697. Whipple, G. H. & Smith, H. P. (1928). Bile salt metabolism: IV. How much bile salt circulates in the body? *J. biol. Chem.* **80**, 697-707.

698. Whiteside, C. H., Fluckiger, H. B. & Sapett, H. P. (1966). Comparison of *in vitro* bile acid binding capacity and *in vivo* hypocholesteremic activity of cholestyramine. *Proc. Soc. exp. Biol. Med.* **121**, 153-156.

699. Wieland, H. & Sorge, H. (1916). Untersuchungen über die Gallensäuren. *Hoppe-Seyler's Z. physiol. Chem.* **97**, 1-26.

700. Williams, C. N. & Senior, J. R. (1971). ^{3}H-cholic acid and ^{14}C-chenodeoxycholic acid kinetic studies in Laennec's cirrhosis: correlation with steatorrhea and pancreatic function. *Gastroenterology* 60, 737 (abstract).

701. Wilson, J. D. (1964). The quantification of cholesterol excretion and degradation in the isotopic steady state in the rat: the influence of dietary cholesterol. *J. Lipid. Res.* 5, 409-417.

702. Wilson, J. D. & Lindsey, C. A. (1965). Studies on the influence of dietary cholesterol on cholesterol metabolism in the isotopic steady state in man. *J. clin. Invest.* 44, 1805-1814.

703. Wilson, J. D. & Reinke, R. T. (1968). Transfer of locally synthesised cholesterol from intestinal wall to intestinal lymph. *J. Lipid Res.* 9, 85-92.

704. Winawer, S. J. & Zamcheck, N. (1968). Pathophysiology of small intestinal resection in man. In *Progress in Gastroenterology,* ed. Glass, G. B. J., Vol. I, pp. 339-356. New York: Grune & Stratton.

705. Windsor, C. W. O. (1968). Gastric secretion following massive small intestinal resection. *Br. J. Surg.* 55, 392 (abstract).

706. Wollenweber, J., Kottke, B. A. & Owen, C. A. (1966). Effect of nicotinic acid on pool size and turnover of taurocholic acid in normal and hypothyroid dogs. *Proc. Soc. exp. Biol. Med.* 122, 1070-1075.

707. Wollenweber, J., Kottke, B. A. & Owen, C. A. (1967). Pool size and turnover of bile acids in six hypercholesteremic patients with and without administration of nicotinic acid. *J. Lab. clin. Med.* 69, 584-593.

708. Wood, P. D. S., Shioda, R. & Kinsell, L. W. (1966). Dietary regulation of cholesterol metabolism. *Lancet* 2, 604-607.

709. Woodbury, J. J., Kern, F. & Palmer, M. (1970). Excretion and enterohepatic circulation of bile acids in patients with diarrhea. *Gastroenterology* 58, 1009 (abstract).

710. Wormsley, K. G. (1970). Stimulation of pancreatic secretion by intraduodenal infusion of bile salts. *Lancet* 2, 586-588.

711. Wright, A. & Whipple, G. H. (1934). II. Bile cholesterol. Fluctuations due to diet factors, bile salt, liver injury and hemolysis. *J. exp. Med.* 59, 411-425.

712. Young, D. L. (1971). The role of micelle-forming properties of bile salts in lipid secretion into bile. *J. clin. Invest.* 50, 101A (abstract).

713. Zurier, R. B., Hashim, S. A. & van Itallie, T. B. (1965). Effect of medium chain triglyceride on cholestyramine-induced steatorrhea in man. *Gastroenterology* 49, 490-495.

Index